Birth Tides

Turning towards Home Birth

Marie O'Connor

An Imprint of HarperCollins*Publishers*

For Colm, Emer and Ruadhán,
who lived to see the day,
and for Nan, who did not.

Pandora
An Imprint of HarperCollins*Publishers*
77–85 Fulham Palace Road,
Hammersmith, London W6 8JB
1160 Battery Street,
San Francisco, California 94111–1213

Published by Pandora 1995
1   3   5   7   9   10   8   6   4   2

© Marie O'Connor 1995

Marie O'Connor asserts the moral right to
be identified as the author of this work

A catalogue record for this book is available from the British Library

ISBN 0 04 440916 8

Printed in Great Britain by HarperCollinsManufacturing Glasgow

Contents

Preface

Perhaps I should point out, firstly, that although the women who appear in these pages are 'real', their names are fictitious. Secondly, where percentages are given, these always refer to the entire sample (N=138), whilst other numbers refer to actual numbers of women.

Every book needs an advocate. Karen Holden, formerly of Pandora, did much to ensure *Birth Tides'* breaking into print. Mary Clemmey, literary agent, acted as its first navigator. Belinda Budge, senior editor, Pandora, steered the manuscript through coral reefs. Marion Steel edited with precision and sensitivity. Her forbearance was remarkable, and her enthusiasm, cheering. Finally, Helen Litton helped with the index.

Encouragement is often what a writer needs most. Sheila Kitzinger has been generous to a fault with hers. Other writers – Suzanne Arms, Barbara Duden, Ivan Illich, Doris Haire, Penny Simkin and Barbara Katz Rothman – gave books, material and advice.

Every manuscript needs readers. Ursula Byrne, tutor midwife, Anne Kelly, independent midwife and Pádraig Ó Snodaigh, publisher and historian, challenged a text not written in stone. Like the others, Máire O'Regan, of the Association for Improvements in the Maternity Services, was generous with her time, and provided material not widely available.

Without the study, there would be no book. The Department of Health, and in particular, its Secretary, Jerry

O'Dwyer, made the project possible, not only by grant-aiding the research, but more crucially, by providing birth registration statistics, enabling me to undertake a national study. Dr John Drumm, former Master of the Coombe Women's Hospital, welcomed the project; his support was a critical factor in ensuring its viability. Bob McCormach of Dublin City University provided the statistical analysis, as well as reading, and re-reading acres of text. These, the outward, visible signs of his input, were equalled, or even surpassed, by the invisible, inward signs, the moral support, the practical advice, given unstintingly over the years. Betty Hilliard, of University College, Dublin, contributed to the sampling and screening phase of the project. Sheila O'Connor, a sociologist, conducted a number of the interviews with skill and sensitivity.

Sometimes a project needs the right person in the right place. Within the health services, many individuals went to considerable lengths to be of help. Seán Fitzgerald, Registrar, General Registration Office, ensured that the ship did not founder on the rocks of bureaucracy. Registration and Community Care staff, particularly public health nurses, identified and traced hundreds of mothers and babies.

Professor James McCormick of Trinity College, Dublin, Evelyn Byrne and Joe Madden of the Central Statistics Office, Professor Brendan O'Donnell, Carmel Hickey and Derek Keyes of the Eastern Health Board, Deirdre Judge and others of the Home Birth Centre, and Rhoda Ui Chonaire of La Leche League, all contributed in their various ways to the project.

Others who played a part were Sr Tríona Harvey, of University College, Dublin, Rudolf Doel of the Institute for Psychosocial Medicine, Mary Daly of Combat Poverty, Brendan Whelan of the Economic and Social Research Institute, Aisling Judge, Dr Stephen Ryan, independent midwives Dolores Staunton and Hannah Barlowe, Drs Seamus Cahalane and Celine Naughten of Temple St Children's Hospital, Eoghan Mac Aogáin of the Linguistic Institute, and Niall O Cearbhaill of Dublin City University.

Without the women who agreed to be interviewed, there

would be no study. Their insights, their honesty, and their time made this book what it is.

Betty Connor kept the home fires burning. Finally, my nearest and dearest provided advice, sympathy, and a welcome respite for what was, all too often over the past four years, a bruising pace. Paul provided valuable material in anaesthesiology. Emer exhorted me to go on, and printed, and photocopied draft after endless draft. Ruadhán did ancillary tasks, having first pointed me in this direction. And Colm listened to streams of consciousness, made dinners and donated the one instrument a writer needs most, a word processor.

Now that its green screen is no longer flickering, thanks.

Foreword
by Sheila Kitzinger

Traditionally women have always drawn on a network of family and sisterhood help in the community before, during and after childbirth. In medieval times when a woman went into labour she called on other women in the neighbourhood to assist her. They were known as God sibs – literally 'sisters in God'. The midwife was one of this group of women. Birth took place at home and women provided the work force, created the choreography, formed the chorus, enacted the initiation ritual and joined together in celebration. Men stayed in the background or left the house. In male language the word 'God sib' gradually became changed to 'gossip'.[1]

Over the past fifty years many skills unique to women, all of which were based on the home, have been steadily eroded and taken over by professionals. Simultaneously women have often lost confidence in their ability to handle the major transitions in their lives. Pregnancy, birth, new motherhood, the menopause, old age and the process of dying have all been medicalized. Expertise is in the hands of doctors and it is they who make the really important decisions. As I did research for my books, *The Crying Baby*[2] and *The Year After Childbirth*[3], I discovered that women are often socially isolated, lack much needed emotional support, and distrust themselves and their own abilities during the important transition experience of new motherhood. The result is confusion, loss of self esteem and often anxiety, panic attacks or depression.

Many professionals see untrained woman-to-woman care as sub-standard and potentially dangerous, basically because it is beyond their control. Birth has been removed from the home to institutions in which the women whom they are intended to serve have no power. Their voices are silenced, and they are conditioned to accept a medical model of birth, and to view it as a pathological process which can only be controlled by the use of technological equipment to stimulate the uterus and by ultrasound monitoring of the fetus under the direction of a medical team. As Ann Oakley points out, 'Technology is never neutral – a thing to be considered in and for itself. Every technology in its mode of development and use will reproduce the power relations of the culture.'[4]

Though it is often taken for granted that hospital must be safer than home, there is no evidence that it is safer for all women to give birth in hospital, and evidence is building that morbidity (harmful side-effects of practice, including illness) in women and their babies is higher in hospital than in home births.[5]

Yet of the women who seek home birth only a very small percentage actually give birth at home. GPs are the gate-keepers to the maternity services in England and Wales. A National Childbirth Trust report[6] reveals that many offer no information and actively prevent women obtaining it by intimidation, 'shroud-waving' and arbitrarily striking them off their lists for daring to insist on giving birth at home.

In England and Wales the home birth rate sank to under 1 per cent until the publication of the Cumberlege report changed government policy and reversed the trend.[7] There are wide regional variations. In many areas of the North of England home birth is rare, while in the Isle of Wight, where midwives are committed to validating women's rights to home birth, it is 8 per cent.

Marie O'Connor's book is a result of a five-year national study of home births in Ireland – the first of its kind in the world. She explores the reasons why women want home birth, the character and backgrounds of the very different kinds of women who decide that home is the best place in which to give birth, their experiences of care in pregnancy, during labour and birth and the physical and emotional outcomes.

Many of these women had previous traumatic hospital births and their distress over what was done to them then was 'etched in the memory'. Antenatal care was sometimes provided on the cattle-market principle, with block bookings of 40 women herded together. Women related how as soon as they crossed the threshold of the hospital they were deprived of identity by having their clothes and personal possessions taken away. They were denied the right to control their own movements, to decline examinations and treatment and, above all, to take their time and follow the rhythms of their bodies in labour. Their most intimate physical functions were dictated and controlled by the hospital. More than half had a compulsory pubic shave. More than half received an enema. These are outmoded, useless and degrading practices which convey the strong message that a woman's body is not her own. Two out of every three women had an episiotomy – the Western way of female genital mutilation. After the baby was born many women had to submit to a restricted and scheduled feeding system, the imposition of which made it clear that the babies belonged to the hospital, not to their mothers.

It is not surprising that these women wanted to have their next babies at home.

Only two-thirds of the women described in this book who chose to have home births would be considered low risk according to one contemporary obstetric 'risk score'. Yet the women encountered few problems, babies were born safely and they were overwhelmingly positive about their experiences. Marie O'Connor shows that the pressure to give birth in hospital had little or nothing to do with the degree of risk run by any particular woman. Twenty-one per cent were 'overdue', with pregnancies of 42 weeks or longer.

Women often had longish labours, too. According to O'Driscoll and Meagher, who invented the system of 'active management', any labour lasting 12 hours or more is prolonged.[8] These obstetricians state that morale drops rapidly after 6 hours, and, 'in geometric rather than arithmetic proportion', deteriorates further after 12 hours. These women, however, and their midwives, coped well with lengthy labours, and did not perceive them as abnormal, though they might be arduous.

It is worth noting that 57 per cent of these women came through with an intact perineum, and only 9 per cent received an episiotomy. The midwives were working under far from ideal conditions, without strong hospital back-up or approval. Continuity of care was sometimes lacking and women sometimes only met their midwife at the end of pregnancy or even when labour started. If midwives working under poor conditions have such good results, what might be achieved when midwifery is acknowledged by obstetricians for the skilled profession that it is, and when midwives can be part of a wider network of woman-to-woman support?

Only when women control the territory in which they give birth can they reclaim childbirth. Only when midwives and mothers build a strong supportive sisterhood which enables women to give birth in their own way, in their own time, and in their own place, can midwifery be reborn.

Sheila Kitzinger
Oxford, April 1995

Time and Tide

Birth is probably the most important thing you're ever going to do in your life [Emily].

It bothers me when I go to a medical conference on the 'management' of labour that no one makes any reference whatsoever to women – as clients, as consumers, or even as patients.[1] Their uterine contractions are 'efficient' or 'inefficient', their cervixes are 'competent' or 'incompetent'; these are the only signs of their existence.

It bothers me when a woman goes to her local health clinic to arrange a home birth that she is asked: 'Have you any consideration for the child?'

It bothers me when I go to a public lecture on obstetrics that an obstetrician tells his largely female audience, many of whom are visibly pregnant, how it is. That childbirth is not now, nor has it ever been, safe, either for mothers or for babies. His colleague at the hospital explains that when God said Eve would bring forth her children in sorrow, what he really meant was that Eve would bring forth her children in pain. He then goes on to describe the benefits, but not the drawbacks, of epidural anaesthesia.[2]

It bothers me when I see birth presented as an acute medical emergency on television. It is always shown as a cross between life-and-death in hospital and a mystery of medical science, with the woman supine on a trolley, her body open to unseen instruments of steel.

Maternity can be a difficult time for women: nobody knows for sure exactly how many women suffer from postnatal depression. Estimates vary hugely.[3] No one knows what causes it. What we do know is that postnatal depression is not necessarily short-term.[4] Some women continue to be distressed for years. Postnatal depression has rarely, in the medical literature, been linked to women's experiences of birth. And women's experiences of the place of birth have seldom been studied.[5]

Home birth raises questions about hospital birth. In countries with a hospital-based system of maternity care, home birth is a demand for an alternative form of care.[6] The management of labour has become so streamlined that once you are admitted to the labour unit, they can tell you when your baby will be born, to within thirty minutes.[7] Labour in excess of twelve hours is regarded by doctors all over the Western world as 'prolonged', and is classified as a complication. The concept of 'progress' is something that has become part of the way doctors think about birth. Caesarian sections are performed in the event of 'failure to progress'.

Birth has become more painful and more frightening. Women are often anxious about what will be done to them in hospital. The procedures used to speed up labour are not intrinsically pleasant. Some women whose labour was accelerated complained, for example, that the drip made their labour too intense, too quickly, that they had no time to get used to it. Routine birth surgery – in the form of an episiotomy enlarging the opening of the vagina – is something else many women particularly object to. Women suspect that in hospital these procedures may not be optional.

Electronic fetal monitoring (EFM) is one of the newer preset programmes now used in many hospitals. These are the machines you see women in labour strapped up to, giving out those electronic bleeps, with the moving graphs on the monitor. This has become the classic television image of birth. The woman is always in bed. She can hardly move. Wires have been inserted up through her vagina attaching an electrode to the baby's scalp. Both the baby's heart-beat and her contractions are monitored, simultaneously. Where fetal distress – the condition monitors are supposed to diagnose – is suspected, the medical response is to get that baby out, fast. Sometimes fetal distress is falsely diagnosed. 'False positives' lead to unnecessary forceps and vacuum deliveries, and to unnecessary Caesarian sections.[8]

Doctors, understandably enough, have become much less willing to take the slightest risk for fear of being sued. Difficult forceps deliveries are becoming a thing of the past. Hospital statistics show a decrease in the number of forceps deliveries, and a corresponding increase in the number of Caesarian sections. When in doubt, doctors say, play safe. 'Playing safe' may mean more Caesarian sections, performed earlier. Playing safe may also mean more routine monitoring. Obstetricians have been sued for not performing a Caesarian section or for not using an electronic fetal monitor.

Epidural anaesthesia is another factor in the growth of Caesarian sections. For 'low-risk' women, having an epidural multiplies the risk of Caesarian by four, according to Frederick Frigoletto of Harvard Medical School.[9] A quarter of all births in the United States are Caesarian sections. Section rates in Europe are fast catching up. And so we come full circle, to a vicious circle. Litigation results in 'defensive' obstetrics. The more doctors intervene, the greater the risk of birth injury. And the more doctors get sued in consequence, the less they will allow women to deliver vaginally. Vaginal breech deliveries – where the baby comes bottom or feet first – are no longer performed in some hospitals. The question we need to ask ourselves is, where will it all end? What kind of birth do we want for ourselves, for our daughters?

Birth by epidural is rapidly becoming the norm. Many women just cannot face the idea of having a baby any more without blocking it out. Epidural anaesthesia used to be restricted to 'exceptional' cases and to first-time mothers. Now, it is on demand in many hospitals, and many women book theirs in advance. These days, the biggest decision facing many pregnant women is whether or not to opt for an epidural in labour. Will we get to a point where the biggest decision

3

facing women in pregnancy is whether or not to opt for a Caesarian?

We are back to the kernel of the argument, the heart of the matter. We need to ask ourselves what is the problem for which an anaesthetic in labour is the solution. And we have glimpsed the answer. Anaesthetic drugs promise a pain-free labour. And women, because they fear birth, because they anticipate pain, because they feel they cannot cope, have bought into this promise. Birth by epidural is one response to the way obstetricians manage birth in hospital. Home birth is another.

༃

The Story of the Research

This is the first time I've talked to anyone about home birth [Máire].

This is the story of women who chose to give birth at home in a country, and at a time, when home birth was virtually outlawed. Some years ago, I set out to do a research project on women's experiences of home births in Ireland. I wanted to find out who was having home births and why, and how they got on. This book is the result of that research. It is an attempt to document these women's experiences, to record everything from their feelings in labour to any complications they might have developed; it is an attempt to answer questions like, is it painful? Is it dangerous?

At the time I began my research little was known about home births in Ireland. But there was some suggestion that home births were on the increase there, just as they were around the world. From the late 1970s onwards, the trend toward home birth was documented in the medical literature in Britain, the United States, Canada, Australia and New Zealand.[10]

Under the 1970 Health Act,[11] local health authorities are

obliged to provide medical, surgical and midwifery services free of charge, at home, to women entitled to them. If the act was to be reviewed, as seemed likely, then something more than the official fiction that all births take place in hospital was needed. The Department of Health, with what appears to be the wisdom of foresight, agreed to fund the necessary research. And the Coombe Women's Hospital, in a spirit of imagination and generosity, decided to support what was, in effect, an independent study.

I ended up with a five-year national study of home birth in Ireland,[12] the first of its kind in Europe or elsewhere, as far as I am aware. Ireland (meaning the Irish Republic here and throughout this book) is a small country, with a population of around three and a half million and a highly developed system of maternity care. It offered 'the best' in micro, on a scale that was feasible to study. It is also a country where people do not move house very often. Mobility levels are low compared to other European countries. People are easier to find. They know their neighbours, which makes it easier to trace families, if they do move.

Finding women who have opted out of the official system of maternity care is not easy. I was fortunate enough to be given access to national birth registration data held by the Central Statistics Office. Taking all the babies (969) listed for five years as out-of-hospital births, I took a random sample, large enough to cover all eventualities. The listing included planned home births as well as BBAs – Born Before Arrivals – unplanned deliveries, which take place in a variety of out-of-hospital settings. The only missing links were planned home births which transferred to hospital, and were subsequently listed as hospital births.

The 480 babies in the sample were then followed up, mostly by public health nurses, to see how many of them were born at home by choice. In most of Western Europe, this kind of research would be difficult, if not impossible, to do. Other countries are simply too big, people move around too much and life is too fragmented. In any other European capital, except Dublin, tracing hundreds of mothers from the birth certificates of their babies would be virtually impossible. Some women had emigrated. A few could not be traced. One woman was dead. Quite a few mistakes had been made in the records. Some listed as home were hospital births. Only one traveller (travellers are reputed to be descended not from European gypsies, but from native Irish families dispossessed in the eighteenth century) came up, and her birth was recorded as a hospital birth. Travellers do not have home births.

Only half of the births were intended to take place at home. The others were BBAs whose mothers did not make it in time, either because they had a short labour, or because the nearest unit was several hours' drive away. They ended up having an unplanned birth at home, or at the side of the road, in a car or an ambulance. A couple of babies were born in doctors' surgeries, and one was born in a police station. If she had not registered the baby, one woman remarked, the state would never have known of his existence.

From the start of the survey an elaborate protocol was laid down in order to maintain confidentiality. I was to get names and addresses only after women had agreed to take part. Some wrote to say how pleased they were that someone, somewhere, was taking an interest in home birth. They saw the study as a way of getting their views across, as paving the way for change. Nearly every woman agreed to take part: the response rate was 97 per cent. Some women had a second home birth during the five years that also came up in the sample, and I eventually ended up with 138 interviews.[13]

Of the four women who refused to take part, two were married to medical practitioners. Their babies had been delivered by their husbands. They felt, with some justification, that their experiences could not possibly be typical. Another refusal came from a former midwife who felt the study lacked credibility, coming, as it did, from one of the country's largest maternity hospitals. The fourth and final refusal came from a woman in a disadvantaged area, who agreed to do the interview, but failed several times to show up.

Before I designed the questionnaire, I went to meetings on home birth where women, and men, told their personal stories. I read whatever I could find, including accounts of home birth written by women. I had discussions with public health nurses, doctors and health officials, civil servants, general practitioners and birth registrars. Above all, I spent time with women, and with midwives, talking about birth, about home birth, about women and the maternity services.

I did twelve thousand miles that summer, interviewing women in their own homes, in kitchens and living-rooms. I did one interview sitting on a rock, on a hot summer's day and another perched on an upturned oil-can by a camp fire, near an ancient abbey.

Interviews lasted about three hours on average. I did over a hundred of them myself, and the others were done by Sheila O'Connor, a former colleague of mine, not a relative. The longest interview was eight and a half hours; we did it in two sessions. Interviews were done in English, with two exceptions; one in French, for rapport, and another in Irish, for ease.

The questionnaire was almost thirty pages long. While it contained quite a large number of open-ended questions, it was fairly structured and extremely detailed. As well as producing statistical information, it was designed to allow women to say whatever they wanted. Not surprisingly, the study generated a huge amount of data, with over seven hundred separate bits of information in each interview. Over eighty thousand items had to be coded, one by one, for the computer. There were times when the sheer volume of data felt insurmountable, when I felt the project was going to shorten my life. But it did result in a body of knowledge on women's experiences of birth at home which is unique.

༄

Birth in Ireland

There are so many midwives but there is this fear. They get no support. The doctors are completely against it. The health board is completely against it. Here, the hospital is forty miles away. There is a demand, and the demand is growing, and there is a lot of antagonism [Thea].

Home birth is not the norm in Ireland, it is the exception. Women who choose home birth are walking on glass during pregnancy. Do you want your baby to be born dead? women are asked, over and over again. In a climate like this, it takes courage to have a baby at home. And where the home birth services have declined to a point where there is no service, or almost none, finding a midwife or a doctor can be a nightmare.

In a country like Ireland, where less than 0.5 per cent of babies are born at home,[14] what makes women do it? Ireland has an international reputation for the quality of its maternity care. One of the oldest surviving maternity hospitals in the world is in Dublin. Babies are not just born in hospital, they are born in large, high-technology units. One of the largest maternity hospitals in Europe is also in Dublin. There are no free-standing birth centres, no midwife or general practitioner units, and few county hospitals or nursing homes where you can go and have your baby.

There has been little research done in Ireland on women's experiences of maternity care.[15] Yet birth is still something most women experience at some time during their lives. As many as 72 per cent of Irishwomen become mothers.[16] In Britain, the figure is slightly higher.[17] And for Irishwomen, birth has the same rarity value that it has elsewhere. Birth-rates are falling more quickly in Ireland than they are in almost any other European country.[18] Maternity in Ireland is hidden from view. Beyond one or two academic theses and dissertations,[19] we know only the fragments, the passing comment in a history of the health services,[20] the fateful episode in the life of a politician.[21] All scribbles in the margins of a history still to be written.

Until this century, birth was unregulated and midwives uncertified. Midwives were employed in each dispensary district, as part of the dispensary medical service set up for the poor.[22] Midwives also practised privately, and their fees were less than those charged by general practitioners.[23] Just as in England,[24] the midwife threatened the practice of the general practitioner. Alleging that 'handywomen', or lay midwives, were responsible for the high maternal death rate,[25] medical practitioners enlisted the support of the Royal College of Physicians in a bid to extend the 1902 Midwives' Act – bringing midwifery under medical control – to Ireland. In 1918, with the help of the Royal College of Physicians, the London-based Central Midwives' Board extended its powers to Ireland. Medical practitioners now had a disciplinary body with which to register complaints against midwives: the newly-appointed board had a majority of medical men.[26] The first step the board took was to invite midwives to register. No distinction was made at first between those midwives who had trained in hospital and those who would now be called 'traditional birth attendants'. The board's requirements were minimal: namely, that the midwife be one year in practice and that she be 'of good character'. Registration was a long drawn-out process, however. Not until 1931 were handywomen brought under control in Ireland.[27]

A hundred years ago, women gave birth at home, and hospital was for the very poor. In hospital women were at risk of 'childbed' or puerperal fever, a deadly kind of blood-poisoning, rife since the seventeenth century. The hands that dissected corpses went on to perform internal examinations, forceps deliveries and other manipulations, unwashed and ungloved. Acute streptococcal infection of the womb followed. Not until the 1880s, twenty years after Ignaz Semmelweis compelled doctors in Vienna to wash their hands in chlorinated lime,[28] did the necessity of hand-washing become accepted by the medical profession. Childbed fever continued to claim women's lives for another fifty years, at least. In 1925, for example, in Ireland, puerperal fever accounted for over half of all deaths of women in childbirth. In Dublin, maternal death rates for hospital and home deliveries in the 1920s and in the 1930s suggest that home was safer than hospital.[29] Similarly in other countries, mortality for women in childbirth was much higher for hospital deliveries than it was for home births.[30]

In 1931, one year after a similar enforcement in Queen Charlotte's in London, gloves were made compulsory for medical students and midwives in the National Maternity Hospital in Dublin. One year later, in 1932, Dettol made its appearance.[31] 1937 saw a dramatic decline in maternal mortality in Ireland, in Europe, and in North America, a decline attributed by some to the introduction of antibiotics, and by others to a sudden and unexplained loss in the power of the streptococcal bacteria itself to cause infection.[32] By 1938, childbed fever, previously the leading cause of death in childbirth for women in Ireland, England and Wales, had dropped into third place.[33]

If childbirth was risky for mothers, it was even more hazardous for babies. Infant death rates were high. Infant mortality was linked to urban poverty, malnutrition and tenement living,[34] and in Ireland, the rates remained relatively unchanged from the beginning of the 1920s until the end of the 1940s.[35] Hospitals encouraged home delivery, admitting only first-time mothers, and those with complications.[36] In Britain, home delivery was considered appropriate for 'normal' confinements, and this view persisted until the 1960s.[37] As late as the 1970s, Scottish general practitioners were issued with a reminder setting out normal medical practice in home deliveries. This memo was reproduced for use in Ireland,[38] together with the guidelines for selecting patients for hospital delivery used in Aberdeen Maternity Hospital.

Irish maternity policy has always reflected British maternity policy, except in areas such as abortion, which is illegal, and certain kinds of prenatal testing, such as amniocentesis, which is not widely available in Ireland. Neither geographical nor political boundaries have been allowed to curtail the development of the professions involved in the delivery of maternity care. In many instances medical examinations can still be taken in either country. This presupposes a common curriculum in medical education. One of the main concerns[39] of the Central Midwives' Board in Dublin was to ensure equivalent standards of training and practice with London to enable Irish midwives to practise in Britain. Midwifery in Ireland continued to be regulated by the British Central Midwives' Board until 1952, when the Irish nursing board, An Bord Altranais, was set up. In the post-war years, hundreds of Irish midwives were trained in, and subsequently worked in British hospitals. Some returned to Ireland to practise.

In those years in rural Ireland, childbirth was still regarded as women's business. A woman was looked after by the district midwife, helped by her mother-in-law and one or two neighbours.[40] A superintendent public health nurse describes district midwifery in rural Ireland as a 24-hour, 7-day week job with 5 midwives for the region, and 25 cases each a year.[41] It worked very well, she said, there were no problems. A former senior public health doctor in the same region agrees:

> You could always ring the hospital and a senior man would come out, with a nurse and an ambulance. It was a service, but there is no service now. People have no choice now but to go to hospital.[42]

In Dublin, the major maternity hospitals ran a district service until the early 1960s, sending out obstetric 'flying squads' if needed. In 1956, 31 per cent of births in Ireland took place at home.[43] Ten years later, home births had dropped to less than 10 per cent. By then, the Maternity and Infant Care Scheme was well in place. A scheme for community-based maternity services to be provided free of charge by the state, it was introduced in 1954.[44] The 'Mother and Child' scheme, to give it its better-known name, allowed for hospital delivery on payment of a small fee. For reasons that have yet to be documented, home births declined in Ireland from the Second World War onwards. Did the fee-paying scheme have the effect of making hospital birth seem the more desirable alternative? One of the mothers I interviewed, Maeve MacElhinney, describes the social changes in rural Ireland in the 1950s:

> When my mother gave birth at home (she came from a well-to-do family in Mayo), people said, 'You'd think she couldn't afford to go to hospital'. It was almost something to be ashamed of.

In the Ireland of the time, what was paid for was what was valued. By 1976, home births had dropped to their current level, 0.5 per cent. It was in that year that Comhairle na n-Ospidéal, a state body with responsibility for structuring consultant posts, recommended that all births take place in hospital, in consultant units. That echoed the 1970 Peel Report in Britain advocating 100 per cent hospital delivery.[45] Four years later, the Maternity and Infant Review Group advised that in the long term, all deliveries should take place 'in maternity units which are fully equipped and staffed at consultant obstetrician and paediatrician level'.[46]

Not only were births taking place in hospital, they were taking place in increasingly large maternity units. In 1966, one third of all births took place in hospitals with more than two thousand births per year. One by one, small nursing homes closed. So did cottage hospitals. Susan Lawlor, another interviewee, speaks approvingly of the cottage hospital where she had her second child:

> There were a lot of older midwives there. No students. A lot of them were married with children. Their episiotomy rate was almost nil.

Ten years later, large-scale institutions accounted for more than half of all births, with a corresponding fall in the number of births in smaller hospitals.[47] Christina Kirwan says you might as well have been at home as be in the small general hospital where she had her first child:

> It wasn't a maternity hospital. The delivery ward was one bed. You had your own doctor [a GP] who came in to deliver you. You knew the nurses. They were the district nurses, some of them. There would always be one or two familiar faces. It was so unrestricted. You didn't meet a stranger from the time you were pregnant to the time you had your baby. There was open visiting. The women used to do things for each other. But that wasn't intervention, it was communal.

Maternity units in general hospitals closed: the delivery ward of one bed was no more. The training needs of any industry can only be met in an environment that is adequately staffed and equipped. In the case of childbirth, with fewer than ten women in every hundred expected to exhibit an abnormality, large numbers of patients are required to present the kinds of complications which medical students need to study. The independent or freestanding general practitioner units, which became a feature of the maternity services in Britain, never developed in Ireland. Irish maternity policy had opted for a consultant model of maternity care. By 1978, 91 per cent of all births in the Republic were taking place in consultant-managed units.[48]

By then, the *active management* of labour in Dublin was well established. Pioneered by Kieran O'Driscoll at the National Maternity Hospital[49] active management is widely recognized as a landmark in obstetrics.[50] A model of consultant care which predetermines the time of birth, it is a programme of obstetrical intervention for first-time mothers, promising doctors a low Caesarian section rate, and women one-to-one attention. The system – which is currently being introduced in a number of American hospitals – has been widely adopted in Britain, resulting in the introduction of new technologies of monitoring and controlling labour.[51]

ᕤ

Identities

They had this idea in the hospital about home birthers – that they lived on the side of a mountain, living a natural life, not accepting any of the norms of society, what they would consider to be 'uncivilized' [Nora].

'They're all vegetarians, aren't they?' one woman said to me. 'They wear handknit jumpers, vote Green, educate their children at home and campaign against nuclear waste.' In a country where home birth is on the margins of maternity care, there is no shortage of stereotypes. Among health professionals in Dublin, the view is that 'they' are always 'well-heeled' and 'articulate' while, outside Dublin, 'they' are all regarded as 'hippies'. Delma, who is one of 'them', says, 'They're all in Greenpeace, against Sandoz [a chemical plant].' I wanted to test the stereotypes.

Women who choose home birth in Ireland tend to be urban, educated, middle-class, married, with children and in their thirties. Not many of them would willingly live on the side of a mountain. Many women see themselves as 'ordinary' married women, as mothers and as wives. Middle of the road, in fact, just like their counterparts in the United States or Australia.[52] Linda remarks that she would have enjoyed the birth more if it had not been regarded as abnormal. And Rita points out that in every other way, she is quite conservative.

Most of the sample group are married, four-fifths to be exact. Only five women were running a household, single-handed, during their pregnancy. At the time of the interview, almost everyone was living in what social workers would call a 'stable family unit'. One woman had been married for 22 years, but 7 is the average. Martina says that though now separated from her husband, the fact that their children were born at home means more than ever: 'We could never really hate each other. We still have the birth of our children bonding us.'

As many as 91 per cent were already mothers. Between them, the women had given birth to 300 children. So the average family size within the group is the almost mythical 2.2. Two-fifths of the group were having a repeat home birth. Kathleen was having her tenth child and Penny her first. Kathleen is in a minority of one.

The group spans two generations. Having this baby at 19 years of age made Trudi the youngest in the group, while at 44, Philomena was more than twice her age. Many women grew up in the 1960s, in the decade of 'alternative' living and 'alternative' health. At the time of the birth, their average age was 30. Fathers tend to be older (with an average age of 33), and between them, they span three generations, from 19 to 59.

14

Four out of five of the women were born in Ireland. Of those who were not, nearly half were born in England. The pattern for fathers is similar. Beatrix says Irishwomen are terrified of giving birth:

> I think that is because they are not as assertive here as they are in Holland. Here the doctor is God. In Holland, it is more of a consumer affair. You can talk to him as an equal. You have your rights.

Comparisons were constantly being made. It is a lot easier to have a home confinement in Germany, Ute says: 'My gynae would have a delivery room, where he would have everything for the delivery.' Nadine, born in South Africa, remarks that in Norwich, in England, lots of women have home births: 'They reinforced my wish to have a baby at home. But Ireland was different.' Claudine, from Geneva, does not think Ireland is different. Ireland is like Switzerland, she says, smiling:

> I really had to fight for a home birth. There are not very many. You are told that you are irresponsible, that you are risking your baby's life.

Nearly half of the group live in their native Dublin, where the maternity hospitals used to operate a district service. Betty says the Iveagh Hospital would send out a crew: 'Me mother delivered many a child in the flats, waiting for the doctor to come.' A third live in the heart of the country, the rest are scattered in towns and villages across Ireland, and most did not know anyone else who had had a home birth.

Women living in cities live in semi-detached houses in suburban estates, or in one of the newer satellite towns. Sometimes they live in red-bricked, terraced houses in the inner city. In Ireland, renting is considered second best, and three-quarters of the group live in privately-owned homes. Only 14 per cent live in local authority houses, and this is in line with national rates.[53] In rural areas, the houses are more varied, with women, and their families, living in old

farmhouses, stone cottages or modern bungalows. A few families live in caravans or mobile homes. Felicity lives in a
covered, horse-drawn wagon, just like the ones travellers used
to live in.

Not everyone in the sample lives in comfort. In rural areas,
particularly, women born outside Ireland are living in what
Irishwomen would regard as hardship. As many as 13 per cent
do not have a bathroom, or an indoor flush toilet. And six per
cent have no facilities of any kind, no electricity or running
water. Not having a phone could cause more problems than
not having a bathroom. Just under half of the group have no
telephone. Living in a deprived satellite town where the public
phones were constantly out of order, Betty's husband had to
cycle a considerable distance before he could locate a telephone kiosk, and the baby arrived before the midwife.

Nearly half of the women have at least some university or
college education and this is in line with women choosing
home birth in other countries.[54] Their partners tended to leave
school earlier. Many women are graduates, like Efa. 'What am
I doing with my degree in geo-physics?' she asks angrily. 'The
washing-up?' But Efa is in a minority. Most women are
working full-time in the home, and they have no desire to do
anything else. Almost half of the group left the labour force
when they got married, became pregnant, or after they had
had their first child. Most have not been in employment for a
number of years.

Nearly a third of the group were involved in work other
than household and child care during pregnancy, half of them
full-time. A number of women work alongside their partners,
doing everything from running a private ambulance company,
to acting as a veterinary surgeon's assistant or running a hair-
dressing salon. Simone and Jacques make baskets, and Thea
and Pietr make farmhouse butter. Elizabeth is an artist. One of
the first pieces of work she ever did, she says, was about
becoming a mother:

> I brought my tape-recorder to the antenatal classes, and
> asked women what they thought the birth would be like.

After the birth I went back, and asked them how things had gone. Some women were very upset, so much so that I couldn't use the data.

Only one woman in the group describes herself as unemployed. Ten per cent of the women had never had a job.

Teaching and nursing are the most popular occupations. Interestingly enough, 11 per cent of the women are or were nursing. Several had trained as midwives. Aylish had worked in a large maternity hospital in Dublin. Deirdre is a physiotherapist in a hospital. Altogether, a fifth of the women had worked in the health sector. Several, like Tara, worked as medical secretaries. This link between having a baby at home and working in the health sector has shown up elsewhere.[55]

Then there are the family connections with midwifery, nursing and medicine. Rachel's mother was a midwife, like Dympna's. Nadine, like several other women, comes from a medical family; as well as her grandfather and her uncle, her father and her brother are both doctors. Nine women in the group volunteer the information that their fathers were doctors.

Only six per cent of the fathers work in the health sector, in medicine, psychiatric nursing or in related areas such as physiotherapy. The men range from engineers, accountants and shopkeepers, to electricians, university lecturers and small farmers. Why there should be so many engineers among them is a mystery, but this may simply reflect the development of engineering itself in recent years. A quarter of them are out of work, higher than the national average.[56] This may be related to the fact that eight per cent dropped out of the labour force, while others were made redundant. Two fathers, previously unemployed, now work full-time in the home.

Statia says that people who have home births tend to be more articulate, more middle-class and more able. Three-fifths of the group are what sociologists would call 'middle-class'.[57] The remainder are split evenly between less well off women, like Betty, who says she went to work at 12 ('If women stood up for themselves more, they wouldn't be treated like cattle'), and women from other countries, like Sonja, who is

German: 'Home birth is to do with having a different attitude, to go back to nature. We are against chemicals.'

Harriet, an Englishwoman whose husband gave up his post as a university teacher, says they were part of the 'alternative' culture. She goes on to describe how a horse-drawn caravan broke down outside their door, when they were living in a Dublin suburb:

> That put us in touch with people here . . . We chose this house because it was very romantic . . . We were very isolated . . . We were very poor . . . My husband wanted to establish a community here. He was interested in alternative childrearing.

Women who are part of the alternative culture tend to be university-educated and to live in rural areas, often in conditions of physical and social isolation and material hardship. Born outside Ireland, quite often, there is nearly always an element of uprooting, of moving between different countries, of contrast between present and former lives in their stories. For example, Penny resigned her job as a computer programmer in London in the 1960s before moving to Ireland, where she subsequently set up a wholefood business.

Looking at the women in the group, it seems, at first, as though they might not have a lot in common. Rosemary lives in a house with a stained-glass conservatory, with a huge garden complete with swimming pool, in a leafy suburb. There is a white Jaguar sitting in the driveway. Her husband is in computers. He has his own company, employing 50 people. Rosemary is now back at college, as a mature student, doing sociology. She has five children, and breast-fed them all until they were three years of age.

Mags lives out in the country, in a small house with a leaking roof, and a husband whose wages have always been low. She has had 8 children in 11 years, and she is now on 15 tablets a day because of her high blood pressure. All her children were bottle-fed. She left school at 15 and works full-time in the home.

Ulrike, who is German, is living with her two children in a tumbledown thatched cottage, without running water or electricity, off a boreen, unmarked and untarred, in an area marketed by the tourist board as 'lakeshore'. Her nearest neighbour lives three miles away.

Ulrike, Mags and Rosemary all planned to have their babies at home.

Like birth by epidural, home birth is a reaction to the way obstetricians manage birth in hospital, to the procedures, to the monitoring, to the Caesarian sections. Women making this choice see themselves, for the most part, as ordinary mothers and married women. But home birth in Ireland is not an ordinary choice. It takes extraordinary courage.

People need to be involved in the decisions that affect them . . . I believe in people being in charge of their own lives [Maude].

The attitude is 'Next, please'. You know nothing, and they won't tell you anything [Netta].

When I was losing the baby at 20 weeks, I went to a doctor. I stood there on his doorstep. I was in pain and he wouldn't see me. 'Not in my lunch-hour,' he said [Patricia].

It's a woman's issue, as I see it. It's been taken out of our control. The medical system has taken control of birthing. The methods they use aren't necessarily best for women [Virginia].

Gynaecologists should admit that home birth is not so unsafe as they make out. They are misleading people to make a few bob [Terry].

Women haven't got the knowledge. They are afraid. They think hospital is the place [Hazel].

✌ 2 ✌

A Sense of Ice

✌

Christina's Story

All I remember is the fear, being left alone in bed. At ten
o'clock, it was shaves and enemas. The following
morning, I woke up as they were wheeling me down to the
labour ward. They wouldn't let me out of bed.

Then they had to catheterize me. That was the kind of
communication there was in there. The nurse said, 'I'll
run the taps'. I didn't know that was supposed to give you
the urge to go to the toilet. I thought, what's she running
the taps for? I started wondering if I was mad . . .

Why was I induced? I was two days over. I didn't have
much choice about it. I was taken in on a Wednesday. At
five o'clock [in the morning], they examined me and put
up the drip. There was no consultation. Everyone was on
a drip. You weren't asked. They broke my waters at six. It
was horrendous . . . The doctor told me to fuck off and
stop screaming.

I asked the sister would she ring my husband, and she
said she would, but she didn't. Things like that, the loneliness . . . I felt very betrayed. The minute I stepped inside
. . . You're told you will be given your own nurse, but the
nurse was a total stranger. And if her shift came to an end,
another nurse came along, another total stranger . . .

They wouldn't let me out of bed. They would let my
sister, who was a nurse, in to see me, but not my husband.

20

The loneliness, the fear, the tiredness, that's all I remember. The stupidity of it. I was freezing cold after she was born. Nobody took a blind bit of notice.

They must have taken away half my insides. The humiliation, the tiredness, the pain . . . There was just no way I was going back to the Iveagh. It was so managed and so contrived.

Christina's first baby was born in a large teaching hospital. The American writer, Suzanne Arms, describes the same feelings of loneliness, fear and tiredness in her book, *Immaculate Deception*.[1] Are women's feelings in maternity hospitals the same the world over?

Deciding to have a home birth is as much a refusal to go to hospital as it is a wish to stay at home. Three-quarters of the group had already had a baby in hospital. Women are walking away from obstetrics, from a system of maternity care that has been characterized as technocratic, managed by technical experts.[2] There are no rosy pictures here of hospital birth, no expressions of thanks to hospital staff for a job well done, like you read in the birth notices of the newspapers. For the majority of women in this study, hospital birth was an experience they simply decided not to repeat. Some women may find this chapter discouraging, if not downright depressing. Some of the stories I was told are awful. I wish I could balance them with stories of sweetness and light. I am sure that lots of women have happy memories of maternity hospitals. Within the group, such happy memories formed no part of women's stories.

In countries where hospital birth is the norm, women who have home births can be expected to have a poor view of maternity hospitals. Maybe women who have positive experiences of birth in hospital simply do not have home births. We do not know. Hardly any research has been done in Ireland on women's experiences of maternity in hospital.[3] Secondly, the time lag between women's hospital births and their interviews may well have resulted in a darker picture of hospital birth. When the wonder of a new baby eventually fades, as it must, do women then go over the birth and reassess their treatment downwards? Research suggests that they do.[4] All we can do here is accept that, within the group, this is how it was for them.

Research shows that home birth is often a response to a bad hospital birth.[5] Anxiety is one of the dominant emotions women express: 'I felt I was only a medium, a quivering mass of flesh,' said Fíona. 'If I wanted a drink of water,' she continued, 'I couldn't even ask for it.' During the course of the interviews, women returned again and again to previous hospital births. Bad hospital births were etched in the memory. For over half of the women I spoke to, it was this experience, in part, that impelled them to have a home birth. What women complained about was the hospital routine, the standard care. 'They have to clear each patient like a package,' Nuala said, 'to get ready for the next one.' Doctors talk half-resignedly, half-ironically about 'sausage factories'. 'It's a conveyor belt,' Charlotte was told by her obstetrician, 'but you'll come out with a live baby.' The image of the conveyor belt suggests the processing of inanimate objects by machine operators. For over thirty years, people have been saying this in the medical journals.[6] To hear women talking about the pain involved – about the indignity and the helplessness, the humiliation and the shame – strips the cliché of its acceptability.

The birth experiences described in this chapter range from the merely unpleasant to the traumatic. At one end of the spectrum there is Carmel, who had what a doctor might call a run-of-the-mill delivery which she found alienating and demeaning. At the other end there is Brenda, who fears her son may become schizophrenic because of the way he was born.

Hospitals are like prisons, Carmel says; they deprive you of your individuality:

The first thing they take away from prisoners is their clothes. They took away my clothes. It was like a jail, you couldn't escape. It was a totally unnecessary interference in a minor matter like clothes. Then when I didn't want to be shaved, it was like I wanted to blow up the hospital. I was totally alien. Nothing was ever explained. I didn't know what pethidine was or an episiotomy. All the explanations were so medical. They were just doing a job. There was no sense of me as a person. And the kitchen was closed when the baby was born, so they refused me tea. They don't even use your name. They always called me 'missus', not Carmel. I hated this, especially as I always use my own name.

Personal belongings are often called 'identity equipment': institutions tend to remove them.[7] Claire, a nurse, pin-points the effect of this: 'The minute you walk in the door, you are stripped of your identity – your clothes and valuables are taken away.' There is the school uniform, there is the prison uniform and there is the hospital gown.

Feeling that as a person she had ceased to exist, Carmel complains that staff failed to explain aspects of her treatment in a way that she could understand. It did not occur to her that she might have been consulted. But Carmel, at least, seemed to have integrated her feelings and could talk about her birth with some detachment. Other women became visibly upset, and I worried for them, for having inadvertently re-opened the wounds of grief and anger, of outrage and bitterness, that kept coming to the surface during their interviews.

Brenda says the hospital caused her 'immense' psychological damage, that it interfered with her life, and with her relationship with her son:

What they do to women in hospitals is obscene . . . I hated it. Something happened to me during that delivery. I became separated from myself, and the baby knew it. I spent four months in bed with him. The baby knew I was detached from him. I couldn't absorb him in the early months like I did the other children. He was nine months or a year before I could feel him absorbed. He desperately needed the touch of human skin. He wouldn't sleep unless he was at my breast. He screamed for hours after he was born. I suffered from severe postnatal depression. He is a damaged child now.

~

Industrializing Birth

Many women feel that, in hospital, instead of individual labours, there is a standard routine for all. There is a stipulated time, they say, an industrial attitude. They see the routine as being for the convenience of staff rather than for the welfare of patients:

> The system is there to suit the hospital, not the mother-to-be. Speeding up the whole process, being made to have the baby the way they want you to. They control it for their convenience, so that there is a quick flow in and out [Fay].

How women feel about their hospital births is related to the way obstetricians manage birth in hospital. How birth is managed will vary from one hospital to the next, just as it will from one country to the next. Sometimes the differences between countries are far less than the differences between hospitals within a single county. Looking at the medical literature around the world, and listening to women talking, it seems that having a baby in Dublin is no different to having one in Durban.

Nadine reports that she was 'hassled' in a hospital in Johannesburg, in South Africa, where she had two births. Both were forceps deliveries, and her second birth was induced. 'When you are in labour you are very vulnerable,' she says. It is a word women use constantly about themselves in the context of hospital birth.

Claudine had her first two children in a private hospital in Zurich in Switzerland. What she has to say sounds all too familiar:

I hated my two births in hospital – the feeling of being taken over . . . They take the measures before they are necessary, the injections, the inductions . . . The process of giving birth is taken away from you.

Looking at the treatment experienced by women in the group who had had a previous baby in a maternity hospital, it became clear that in this respect at least, they had a lot in common. Many women complained of births that were 'managed' or 'contrived'. Until recently, having a baby without first being given an enema was not allowed. Neither was it possible to give birth with one's pubic hair intact. In some hospitals, of course, it is still not possible.[8] Half of the women I spoke to had this routine preparation for labour. None of them showed any enthusiasm for it. 'Enemas and shaves should be done away with,' says Joan. Sheila Kitzinger, in her book, *Ourselves as Mothers*, says that in giving a woman an enema in labour, the hospital is taking control over an intimate bodily function. And pubic shaving, she says, is yet another ritual, part of the making of a compliant patient.[9]

❧

Speeding Things Up

In hospital for her second baby, Charlotte heard the staff say something about doing an ARM:

I didn't know what it was. I asked the nurse. She just went and got the doctor, without saying anything. The doctor came in. He thought I was complaining about something. He explained it by saying, 'Your baby may be in stress'.

He could have told her that they wanted to do an 'amniotomy', to puncture the sac of amniotic fluid her baby was lying in. Since the middle of the eighteenth century, physicians have known that rupturing the membranes induced labour.[10] It is done by inserting an obstetric instrument, not unlike a crochet hook, into the vagina. In some hospitals, it is done as a matter of course to bring on or speed up labour. It is also done to examine the colour of the liquid around the baby. If the waters are stained with meconium – a product of the baby's bowel – this is seen as an indication that the baby may be in distress. Over 50 per cent of the women in the group had their waters broken on a previous birth. Like many women, Angela complains about the way it was done:

> I was only 19 at the time. The Master [the obstetrician appointed as chief executive] was in a suit and tie. He just came along with these scissors . . . I was left sitting in a wet bed for two hours. It was outrageous, very embarrassing.

Geraldine says they forced her to have her waters broken even though she did not want them to:

> I went in as a public patient. I was eight centimetres dilated when I went in, and they still had to do an amniotomy. I raised the matter and I was told that, if you have your baby in hospital, these are the safety procedures. It threw me off balance completely in my labour. There was this feeling of not being in control. I felt very violated. You've got no say whatsoever.

Tríona, an architect, also felt she had no choice in the matter. The doctor told her the baby was deteriorating:

> I was crying as he was trying to rupture the membranes. They don't like anything emotional. I was very upset. I'd wanted a natural birth. I felt it was an invasion of my body. I felt raped. It affected my physical relationship with my husband.

Psychologically, Tríona says, it probably affected her for about two years. Having one's vagina forcibly penetrated with an object is recognized legally as a form of rape. It is not difficult to see how a woman could feel violated by such an action, regardless of the medical intention or the hospital setting.

Many of these 'interferences', as women called them, like inducing or accelerating labour, are done routinely. Another way of bringing on or speeding up labour is by dripping oxytocin directly into the vein. The effect of pituitary gland extract on the human womb was described by physicians at the turn of the century, but it was not until 1955 that it was produced in synthetic form as oxytocin.[11] Being 'thrown in at the deep end' is how women often describe its effect on them. It makes the contractions of the womb both more frequent and more intense.[12] Many women echo Nuala's complaint about the severity of the drip:

> It won't be painful, they said, it will be slow . . . I had an abominable contraction . . . Every inch of me left the bed with the pain . . . It got so bad I tried to pull it [the drip] out.[13]

Catherine was having her first baby in a small maternity unit in a large general hospital. She makes the drip sound like one more nail in the cross:

> It was awful, the interference. I had no complications. I have no proper memory of it. They removed my brain. I was afraid to think about it afterwards. You were in a constant state of tension. The horror of the drip . . . It was one unmentionable horror after the other, as if you weren't nervous enough.

᪥

Birth on Schedule

Complaints about forced births were common. Being able to mark off the day on the calendar, knowing that you are scheduled for induction, changes everything. Cecilia was induced on the day the baby, her first, was due:

> It was because of my height and the size of my shoes. I'm not very tall. They thought I [the baby] was too small [for its age in weeks]. The doctor was just back from his holidays. It was a Friday, and he just wanted to get through them for the weekend. It was a production line . . . You're not in a position to argue. The drip was too hard and too fast. I got pethidine. I had hallucinations. There was no gap in the contractions. They [the staff] were busy. They wouldn't let husbands in. My husband was holding the drip bottle for another woman in the corridor . . . They kept telling me to push. I said, 'I am pushing', but I wasn't. The doctor said, 'I am going to give you an injection, and when you wake up, you will see your baby'. I was pushing for an hour and twenty minutes at that stage. That's why they used the forceps. I couldn't push because of the drugs. It was a lift-out forceps, a Barn's forceps, I think it's called. It's all very hazy because I was so drugged . . . He had an Apgar score of eight, so he was put into an incubator.

Induced babies occasionally end up in an incubator. A newborn baby's Apgar score is assessed immediately after birth, based on the child's appearance, its pulse, its breathing and its overall condition and behaviour. The score can vary from 0 for babies in extremely poor condition, to 10 for infants in particularly good shape.

Not many women want to be induced. Ann Cartwright, in her study of induction in Britain, found that only one in every three women felt that they had a choice in the matter.[14]

୬

Having an Episiotomy

'You know when you cut a chicken?' Nuala asks me. 'I literally heard the sound of flesh being cut.' Middle-class women use the medical term 'episiotomy': less well-off women talk about being cut. In English, there is no other word available to us for this form of birth surgery. Again, like the Greek word, *amniotomy*, it distances women from the often painful reality of their own embodied experience. Not upsetting the hospital routine is what mattered, Nuala says. As long as you are safe and the baby is safe, nothing else counts, she reckons, as far as staff are concerned:

> I didn't want an episiotomy. The midwife's attitude was, 'I'll do it anyway, just in case'. It's not down to what's right for the woman, it's down to the system, the whole thing . . . Hospital is clinical. Your mind is taken from you. You don't have a say.

Episiotomy involves enlarging the opening of the vagina by anything up to several inches, cutting towards the rectum or to one side or the other through the tissue with a pair of obstetric scissors. This surgical technique was developed in Dublin in the Rotunda Hospital by its second Master, Fielding Ould, who wrote about it in 1742.[15] Some obstetricians have suggested that as a routine it should be abandoned as useless.[16] But it certainly has not gone out of fashion. Catherine says her experience in hospital changed her attitude towards giving birth:

> It was a degradation. It damaged my relationships with my husband and with my children. I went off sex for years. I didn't know why. The episiotomy was 100 per cent the worst. They cut me. I had to have stitches inside and out. I couldn't push the baby out. [She had a forceps delivery.] It

was deadly damaging . . . Birth in hospital is like a conspiracy of silence. It's unbelievably painful.

Catherine would agree with Sheila Kitzinger's description of episiotomy as a form of 'female genital mutilation'.[17] It can result, later, in painful sex, and this is recognized in obstetrics textbooks. Two out of every three women I interviewed had this form of birth surgery.

Surgery of any kind requires stitching, and episiotomy is no exception. Doctors are inclined to smile, resignedly, when they hear women complaining about stitches. It is as though, like sausage factories, they have become part of the familiar folklore of birth, an archetypal feature of the stories. Laura says her stitching was 'horrendous'. Ursula, an antenatal teacher, having her first baby, almost apologizes for bringing it up:

I had six stitches without an anaesthetic. It was dreadful. I wouldn't make a fuss about it only I know it happens to lots of women. The local anaesthetic had worn off – it was about an hour after the birth – they just didn't check.

She had an enema, shave, amniotomy, oxytocin, pethidine (a painkiller), gas and an episiotomy. 'The birth was absolute hell,' she says.

The net effect of all these procedures, Tara says, is that going into hospital to have a baby is like going in to have something removed. Giving birth has become a medical routine: 'It's the same procedure as an operation.' Frances, a former nurse, is angry about what she sees as the attitude of obstetricians:

Mothers are supposed to know nothing about it. There was no process [of giving birth]. They take away your honour as a woman.

What if you want the process without the procedures? Niamh was having her first baby at 18 in a large teaching hospital:

I had a fierce battle in Green Street. I had to fight to even be allowed to stand up when I got a contraction. They wanted to give me gas, and that monitor, the one they put on your stomach. I didn't want it. I didn't want an enema or my waters broken . . . They kept firing my husband in and out. At one stage, they called in the wrong husband. This fellow came in, and said, 'She's not my wife', and I said, 'That's all right, he's not my husband'!

They wanted to give me an episiotomy. When I saw them arriving in with the stirrups, these leather straps on a chain like a dog's lead, I said, 'No thanks'!

Niamh had read loads, she said, during her pregnancy, out of the library: 'The last thing you want to do in labour is to fight.'

&

Rosemary's Delivery

I was induced on Rosemary. She was 11 days over . . . The drip fell out and it went into the tissue. My hand all swelled up. My labour stopped. My veins collapsed. They had to try a few places before they could get the needle back in. It was a nightmare . . . The drip made it too hard too fast. You were launched halfway into labour before you'd even started, with no time to get used to the pain . . .

They had me on a monitor, one of the ones they put up through you. I found the monitor terribly uncomfortable. I couldn't move. They made me lie on the bed from eleven o'clock when they broke the waters to five past ten when she was born. Telling me what I ought to do . . . They gave me no information at all on the labour or on the baby. The heart slowed down at one stage. The machine broke down but they brought in another one. They also used one of those ear trumpets.

During the birth I got confused. I didn't know my own name. I got cold. I think I must have gone into shock. They brought one of the head guys down to see me. The cubicle seemed to be full of people. My husband was the only person I wanted to be there and they wouldn't let him in.

I had an epidural. I couldn't push. I couldn't feel anything. I had to have a forceps. It was a Barn's forceps. It was all wrecked. I felt tired and depressed after it. Now I always tell everyone not to have an epidural. If I'd thought about it, it stands to reason. If you're numb from the waist down, you're not going to be able to feel any pushing sensations. But I didn't think about it. If I'd known, I wouldn't have had it [Florence].

Drips fall out occasionally, and veins have been known to collapse. Machines break down. These things happen. In other ways, Florence's story has all the hallmarks of what we have come to associate with a bad birth: being routinely induced because the baby is x days over, with oxytocin making her labour too hard too fast; the discomfort and enforced immobility of being wired up to an electronic fetal monitor, having first had her waters ruptured in order to get an electrode recording the baby's heartbeat clipped onto his head, and wearing another device belted around her stomach registering her contractions; being surrounded by numerous strangers; not being given any information on the baby, or on the 'progress' of the labour; not being allowed to have her husband with her; being given an epidural without first being told she might have to have a forceps delivery as a result; being told what to do; feeling that she was just another body being put through the system. Florence was having her first baby at the age of 22 in a large teaching hospital in Dublin: 'I was disgusted at the way I was treated.'

჻

Doing It Their Way

Medical 'interventions', of course, are almost always referred to as 'procedures'. The word *procedure* suggests that not only is this how it is done, but that this is the only possible way of doing it. There may be a dispute about an action, there can be none about a procedure.

The issue of control or, rather, the lack of it, surfaces again and again in women's accounts. Nuala explains why she had oxytocin even though she did not want it: 'I had a stupid attitude, trying to please people, not making waves. It was the way I was brought up.' Women came to a realization of their own powerlessness in different ways. Sometimes it was because hospital staff neglected to consult them. Sometimes they found that their clearly expressed wishes were ignored. Being in hospital reminded Tríona of being in school, when you were constantly in the power of others:

> It was like school. Everyone used to hang their washing on the radiators to dry. Everything used to be whipped off before matron arrived: 'Good morning, girls. Are you behaving yourselves?'

Indignation occasionally surfaces: 'We were all married women, not fifth years,' Frances, a former nurse, says tartly. Helena evokes the image of the 'good' patient: 'If I was in hospital again, I would be quite demanding, a "difficult" patient. If you're a "good" patient, you get walked on.' Clearly, the 'good' patient is like a 'good' girl, docile, submissive, obedient, and less than adult.[18]

Women occasionally complained about inflexible hospital routines. Having to get up at six o'clock in the morning, being woken to have your temperature taken, or to be asked if you want a sleeping tablet, these are minor complaints. More serious was the complaint from one woman in five of lack of information, either on medical procedures, or on the progress of her labour.[19] Tara's view is that doctors don't tell you things:

> The first time I was in hospital, they caught me reading my notes. The second time, I was caught reading them again, and after that they wouldn't let me handle them at all. They treated us like small children.

Within the group, the view is that maternity hospitals fail to respect women's right to decide for themselves in labour. 'When I was having my second baby,' Catherine recalls, 'I went to see the Master. His attitude was, "Do what you're told". As if I was six.' Medical ethics require that doctors respect a person's autonomy.[20] This was not Laura's experience.

> They set down the procedures; if you didn't want them, you were made to feel you were rocking the boat. You must succumb, in general. If you don't, they won't be as pleasant to you. If you're 'Yes, doctor, no, doctor', fine, but if you have reservations, the voicing of opinions is difficult. It's an intimidating situation. Once you sign in, you become part of the system. A lot of it is out of your hands.

Four out of five women in the sample believe this. Part of the admissions drill in Irish maternity hospitals involves being asked to sign a 'blanket' consent form, authorizing the hospital to carry out whatever treatment obstetricians deem to be necessary. Vicki describes how she refused to sign hers:

> They gave me a form to sign, consenting to everything. I gave it back to them. Then they put another form on my belly. I scribbled on it.

Women talk about lack of freedom, lack of choice, and lack of control. 'Doctors play God and carry out procedures against people's wills,' Jacqueline, a Muslim woman, observes. This is how it is seen within the group. 'You were at the mercy of whoever was on at the time. It was for them to decide what you needed.' More than anything else, this is why women feel such a sense of grievance in relation to their hospital births. How forceful can you be in labour? You are not in any condition to fight when you are in labour, Patricia maintains: 'It's your whole centre of gravity down there, isn't it? The pelvic muscles?' What happens if you assert yourself? Some women believe it only leads to confrontation. Tríona sees the hospital as a battle-field:

The hospital environment is hostile. You feel you're under siege, under attack. You are suspicious, defensive. It's intimidating. If you ask a question, you are made to feel [you're being difficult].

A number of women – 16 per cent – complain of hostility or retaliation on the part of hospital staff. It was usually verbal: the incident related by Rachel is the only one of its kind in the group:

The night I was in, there were 13 other women in the labour ward. They were very, very busy. I was young and naive. When you're in labour, you couldn't be more vulnerable . . . They gave me a soap-and-water enema. Imagine, in this day and age, a soap-and-water enema! I didn't want it, but they insisted. Maybe if I'd argued more forcibly . . . There was a student there. He kept on testing the fetal heart . . . They do a rectal exam in there. It was painful. They went on and on doing them. They just came along and rolled me over. I felt like a big sow.

It was a nightmare. When I wanted to lie down, they wanted me to be up. When I wanted to be up, they wanted me to lie down . . . My legs were in stirrups. This doctor came in. He washed his hands. He put on gloves. He didn't address me. He didn't look at me. I wasn't screaming or anything, but I must have been shouting. He said, 'Would you stop this behaviour, Mrs Roberts? You're disturbing the other patients.' And all the time he kept on and on trying to break the waters. I'd wanted no interference.

Early on in the labour, I was offered pethidine. I said no. I was offered it again, later. I said yes. They kept on sending Seán out. 'Mrs Roberts,' the nurse said, 'you're disturbing the whole labour ward.' The midwife told me to push. 'Push, push,' she said. 'You're ready.' 'I'm not going to push 'til Seán's here,' I said. That was the only thing I could do. I knew they hated me.

Then they did a routine episiotomy. I didn't want a

routine episiotomy. The stitching was done by another male doctor. He was rough. I was strapped up. At one point, he said 'It can't be that sore, after having a baby. Can't you bear a few stitches?' He was trying to take out these cotton wool swabs. I suppose I was shouting. I said, 'You're very rough.' He said, 'All right, they can stay there.' I didn't believe him, I thought he was just saying it. Three days later, they were still in . . .

Leaving cotton swabs in deliberately is unheard of, but in every other way Rachel's story is fairly unexceptional. She was having her first child at the age of 21 in the teaching hospital where she had trained as a midwife. Afterwards, she says, she had nightmares about being in hospital, about being out of control: 'Maybe I was extra sensitive, but I don't think so.'

~

On Being Examined Internally

Many women loathe being examined internally. Vaginal examinations have been described in the medical literature as being dehumanizing.[21] Rectal examinations are an alternative, but not, as far as Emily is concerned, a very good one: 'I'm very private about my body,' she says. 'To put it crudely, I don't like everyone looking up my ass!' Being examined in this way, repeatedly – as often as every two hours in some hospitals – the practice begins to take on the appearance of torture.

Within the group there were plenty of complaints about how internal examinations were done. Internal examinations are often carried out by male doctors in a deliberately impersonal way, it has been suggested, to protect themselves from any suggestion of sexual impropriety.[22] It is precisely this refusal to make interpersonal contact when the nature of the physical contact is so invasively intimate that women find so unacceptable. 'The internals were the worst,' Una says. 'It's the feeling you get in hospital. They wouldn't even look at you. It's embarrassing.' Women do not understand that this may be a defence mechanism. Instead, they feel depersonalized and humiliated by being examined in a way that reduces them to just another vagina, or rectum.

❧

On Being Given Mind-altering Drugs

Pethidine, or demerol, a synthetic opiate, is the only pain-killer used routinely in labour in many hospitals. If, as a result of all these medical procedures, labour is made more painful, then the need for painkillers must be exacerbated.[23] Over 40 per cent of women in the group had pethidine on a previous birth; a small number related how pethidine had actually been forced on them against their wishes. Deborah, a former nurse, recalls being turned over in bed for an injection:

> I wasn't asked did I want it. The nurse would just come along, turn me over, and give it to me. There should be more communication. Even if it was hard going, I'd rather be asked.

Being turned over for a shot of pethidine is not too different from being rolled over for repeated rectal examinations. There is the same feeling of being an inert object, a sense of being reduced to 'a thing without a head', as Betty described it.

❧

Not Being Free to Move

Freedom begins in and with the body. Being confined to bed against their will during labour was a recurring complaint among women:

In the hospital I had to make excuses to go to the toilet so I could move around. I thought I'd have the baby in the toilet [Lena].

It can heighten the stress of labour. 'You can't cope with pain lying on a bed,' Joan says. 'It was a nightmare, having to lie there in bed when you had backache,' Betty recalls. Other women with backache labours say exactly the same thing.

Physical confinement does not necessarily come to an end with the first stage of labour. They should not dictate to mothers how to give birth, Joan maintains: 'You should be free to stand up or sit down if you want to.' Women complained over and over again about being forced to deliver on their backs, in what is knows as the 'lithotomy' position. Patricia describes how, in the height of labour, she struggled in vain with staff to stay crouched:

In hospital you feel like an artefact. You've lost control. Your dignity is taken away from you. What they do is very humiliating. I was crouched down, and they kept on trying to get me to lie on my back. It put awful pressure on my spine. I think it injured my back having to deliver in that position.

To Niamh, stirrups looked like 'leather straps on a chain like a dog's lead'. In her case, they were to be used for an episiotomy. Other women were forced to give birth in this way. They found it indecent. 'Births with your legs up in stirrups in hospital are very degrading,' Jacqueline says. 'It's like being a prisoner.' The use of stirrups in childbirth has been described in the medical literature as a threat to women's body image and identity. [24] But it is much more than a mere threat; it is a form of physical restraint. Frances, a former nurse, feels that in hospital her right to bodily integrity was violated:

Hospital was an intrusion on me as a woman. They do everything to see to it that it is a confinement. You really are confined . . . ! Your legs in stirrups . . . You are a prisoner . . . I felt torn to pieces physically after the two in hospital. I felt that my body wasn't my own.

ॐ

Keeping Fathers Out

Being separated forcibly while in labour from your partner is one of the major complaints women have. A quarter of the group report that there were difficulties in arranging for their partners to accompany them in labour. Women found such enforced separation extremely threatening.[25] In two out of three such episodes, hospital staff refused to allow fathers to remain with their partners. Leslie, a teacher, had a protracted battle with staff over the matter:

The first time, I didn't have my husband with me. I remember they actually said to me, 'Be quiet, or we'll leave you on your own.' With the second, I asked for my husband and they said that husbands weren't allowed. I said that if that was going to be the case, I wasn't going to go into the labour ward. I was sitting on this chair at the time. There was consternation. They brought the matron, and he was allowed in, eventually. You have to be able to stand up for yourself, or they bully you.

Being left alone in labour is something many women dread. A number of women, like Catherine, describing emotionally difficult births, mention that they were left alone in labour: 'I was just mentally switched of. I was left on my own. I freaked.' It is a complaint that surfaced in the literature over a quarter of a century ago.[26]

At home fathers act as general go-fors and chief boilers of water, as personal bodyguards and principal back-rubbers. In hospital, even when they are present, men's role can appear to be very restricted.

Even though my husband was there, he had to wear a paper gown as if he were just the biggest germ in the room. Then afterwards he was left standing outside the door for two hours. They were supposed to be tidying me up but there was nothing to be done, really [Lelia].

The alternative to being left alone in labour, as Nora saw it, was to have your husband with you. What is important, she says, is that he is not asked to leave before an internal examination: 'It's the break of contact which leaves you isolated.' She took it for granted that her husband could accompany her into the delivery room, but that was unheard of in the hospital at the time:

There was a whole lot of verbiage, a lot of abuse, and he was bodily lifted and thrown out. And the consultant said we were itinerant people with no records. He was very abusive. My husband told him he'd sue him and sue the hospital for everything they had.

After the birth, it took her husband nine months to relate to their son: 'It was then that I realized how central the birthing process is.'

꒳

Taking the Baby Away

With the advent of bonding theory, many women now believe that there is a critical period after birth, which is vital for mother-child attachment.[27] A quarter of the group were forcibly separated from their newly-born babies. Women found such enforced separation deeply upsetting. Patricia describes how her child was taken away from her:

It was like a concentration camp . . . The paediatrician said it was better for the mother to get a good night's sleep, they said. I cried all night until I got her back at six o'clock in the morning. And she'd sucked her wrist so much you could see the mark.

To be separated from the baby you have just pushed out into the world goes against the grain for many women. As a grievance within the group, it ranks only with being separated forcibly from your partner during labour. Listening to Nuala, it is difficult to know where her anguish ended and her daughter's began:

> They put her in a room. She cried and cried and cried . . . The following morning, the nurse said, 'You're going to have your hands full with that one. She's been crying all night.' Her face was contorted. Her mouth went from ear to ear. The reddishness and blueness had gone down, so you could really see the broken veins. She was like an oul' granny. There was anguish written all over her . . . She'd gone through the process of dying.

Women sometimes fear that they will be given the wrong baby. It is an anxiety that is not totally groundless,[28] although the odds against it are extremely high. Separation can also lead to other fears and anxieties, as Charlotte reveals, whilst highlighting not just the difficulties of communication but also her own powerlessness in hospital:

> I asked the nurse was my baby all right. She said 'She's over there.' She didn't answer the question. So I thought, maybe there was something wrong with her.

This was the prelude to a succession of difficulties created by the separation of mother and child.

> She was small, so they put her in an incubator. They said to Bob, 'Your little baby is very tired.' I felt I'd missed the experience of holding her [after she was born]. They gave her glucose. At eleven o'clock, I wanted to feed her, but

they said, 'Get some rest. We're going on our tea-break, and we'd have to be with you, so we'll give her a little more glucose.' When Bob came back at lunch-time, I still hadn't fed her.

The practice of separating mother and child makes breast-feeding more difficult and a number of women criticized the practice of routinely giving babies glucose. Women also felt that the hospital practice of scheduling feeds, allowing mothers to feed their babies only once every three or four hours, was counter-productive. Finally, women sometimes complained of not being given enough help and guidance with breast-feeding.

☙

Among Strangers

'You're a number,' Joan says. 'You take your turn. I don't like it.' Nobody likes it. After powerlessness, depersonalized care is the second most common grievance within the group. For Catherine, a set designer, the experience of being discounted as a person began on admission. She was indignant at the idea of being 'asked to wait at a desk, and not to be told for whom and for how long'. It is a complaint that less well-off women never made. Women who are better off expect more from the system than those who are not: 'The care is utterly impersonal,' Catherine observes. To be treated intimately by someone you do not know, by someone you have not been introduced to, offends her sense of what is acceptable, of what is proper. In many hospitals, an internal examination is performed on admission to determine whether or not labour has begun.[29] Being looked after by strangers makes preliminaries difficult.

Taking no notice, paying no attention is part of how women experienced their care from hospital staff. Betty says that, if you have a complication, you are much more interesting than if you are just the assembly line:

If you differ from the other patients, you get loads of students around you, but they never explain anything to you. They will talk to the doctor or to the sister, but not to you . . . It is very impersonal. You are just another customer.

Half of the group felt that hospital staff were unwilling to communicate with them. Like others, Tríona found the experience of hospital humiliating: 'They don't regard your state of mind as important – the less you use it the better!' A number of women were dissatisfied because hospital staff refused to believe them at a critical moment. Cynthia says they were cleaning shelves instead of paying attention to her: 'They wouldn't believe me that I was ready to deliver my baby. They left everything to the very last second.' Like stitching episodes, this is one of the archetypal complaints made by women in labour.

Part of why women see it like this is because of the routine processing of their bodies in labour. At ten o'clock, it was shaves and enemas, Christina said at the beginning of this chapter. Women who are public patients (see page 52) are more likely to see maternity hospital care in this way. But it is a view that is shared by other women. It is rooted in the way staff are seen to relate to women having a baby, in the way the hospital is seen to be organized.

Women were particularly critical of the shift system, where they felt themselves to be at the mercy of whomever happened to be on duty at the time:

It all depended on the sister who was on at the time. There were three teams, each on an eight-hour shift. One team was into natural childbirth . . . and one was into mechanized childbirth [Aylish].

For many women, the idea of being looked after by total strangers in the height of labour is a nightmare. For women whose labours do not fall within a single shift, it means being looked after by a succession of midwives. It means that whatever relationship has been built up between a woman and a midwife comes to an abrupt end with the clock. And it means, as Tara said, that 'you have to keep telling them, to keep arguing.'

To Chrissie, the hospital where she had her first baby reminded her of the manufacturing company where she had got her first job:

> It was like a factory, with shift workers and no communication between them. I thought, 'If I keep calm and don't cause trouble, it will be better.' But I think now I'd have been better off if I'd screamed. I might have got more attention.
>
> I told them when I went in. I said, 'Tell me when to push, when the time comes.' It was my first baby. I didn't know what to expect. They had this monitor on me, and the nurses went off and a different set came on. They said the baby's heart was in distress, but I was just waiting, trying to hold me legs in . . . They nearly gave me a section. They were going to use a forceps. I heard the doctor saying, 'We could nearly have got this one with an episiotomy.' And I said, 'Am I supposed to start pushing?' He said yes, and I said, 'It's a pity you didn't say that earlier.' I could have laughed. They actually had the forceps in at the time. And I'd told them to tell me when to push. I hated the hospital. It was a production situation. You were just a number. It was off-putting.

Middle-class women are likely to interpret such a disregard for them as individuals in gender terms. This is how Sinéad, a former teacher, sees it:

> It's the whole system in hospital, the way it treats people. I think the way they treat women is dreadful. They talk over you. You are a thing. I was wired up to a machine in hospital, and it was so loud, it was driving me crazy. But they take no notice. They just tell you to shut up and get on with it, like everybody else.

Ellen hints at the consequences of being reduced to an extension of the machinery:

> They don't usually inform you, do they, if they're going to give you an injection or whatever? They just come along and do it. In hospital, doctors and nurses talk to each other, but not to you. There isn't a lot of communication. They don't tell you what they're doing. You are an object to them. You're being used.

Sometimes, listening to women talking, it is difficult to disentangle the threads of powerlessness from those of depersonalized care, to distinguish between lack of communication and lack of control. Lelia is explicit about the connection:

> You are treated in hospital like a lump of meat. It was the procedures in hospital that I didn't like. The doctor not talking to you. Talking to the nurse as if you couldn't hear when you were in labour. You really become this medical object, and it's all about the production of a child.

Many women complained that staff were rude, insensitive, or just plain uncaring in their treatment of them. In hospital, Celia says, they do an internal when it suits them, regardless of whether or not you are having a contraction. This is a recurring complaint within the group. Women find this kind of treatment incomprehensible. They do not understand that Western medicine was built on the idea of the body as a machine.[30]

Medicine lacks transparency. One of the unwritten rules in hospital is do not burden the patient with medical information she does not need. Women do not understand this, and they are likely to interpret the withholding of information in ways which may surprise doctors. For women who are less well-off, not being informed is a mark of low esteem, a measure – as far as they are concerned – of how they are seen by hospital staff. 'They didn't think enough of me to tell me the afterbirth had broken off,' Nuala says, bitterly. Florence also attributes the fact that staff omitted to tell her what had happened to the fact that she was not important enough:

> I'd had sixteen stitches. I was torn inside. They didn't tell me. My womb could have come out, and they wouldn't have told me . . . They treat you like an animal.

৵

Doctor-induced Damage

Sometimes the decision to have a home birth could be triggered by a single experience. In Jean's case, it was the experience of a miscarriage, a baby who lived for two hours:

> I had a miscarriage at five and a half months. It was traumatic, harrowing. There wasn't a lot of sensitivity. It was frightening. I found it clinical. There wasn't a lot of information. I would have liked to have been brought into the consultant's room and told this is why he didn't live, but I wasn't. I've never told my children about it. My husband and I never discussed it. I never told anybody about it until now. It was a boy.

Jean is complaining of lack of information, of lack of communication. Betty believes that in her case there was negligence:

> There was neglect. They thought it was the afterbirth coming. They didn't know it was twins. It nearly broke me up. One of them should have lived.

She gave birth to twins at 32 weeks: they lived for a day. Later, the doctor told her he was sick of women coming in crying. Had Betty been told why the twins did not live, then her view might have been different. She is the second mother in the group to have given birth to twins who did not survive. The other is Felicity, who had an unattended birth, and

46

whose story is told in Chapter 7.

Sometimes it seems that, like an advertizement on the wall of a Pentecostal church in Dublin bearing the legend, 'All Human Life Is Here', the group encompassed almost every possible maternity experience. In Delma's case, her baby survived:

> I was a private patient. I went in at eleven at night. The consultant didn't come until eight in the morning. I was in labour all night. He just put me out and hauled him out. It was a high forceps. They never told me there was anything wrong with him, but they had him in an incubator for two weeks. He was blue. It was lack of oxygen. They left me too long in labour. He's been in Rockhill [a residential centre for young people with disabilities] now for three or four years. He's one of the better ones. He didn't speak 'til he was seven or eight. It affected his motor function as well.

She said she would not have had another child had she not been able to have a home birth. Her personal tragedy – unique within the group – bears witness to one of the dilemmas facing obstetricians. Had Delma sued, her case might have been fought on the basis that her obstetrician should have intervened earlier, and that he should have performed a Caesarian section.

ॐ

Deborah's Story

Deborah, a former nurse, opted for private medical care on her third baby, having gone to hospital as a public patient for the first two. It was supposed to be the perfect birth:

> When I went in, the nurse examined me. An hour later, the gynaecologist came. He put up a drip which he said

was glucose. A couple of minutes later, I could feel myself going. I went out and came to when the contractions were at their worst. I was on my own in the labour ward. They had to wake me up for the birth. The nurse put her hand over my mouth and pinched my nostrils to get me to push. I thought I was choking. I started to move my arms and legs in the air. The gynaecologist came in and asked me if I would like to go to sleep. I said yes, of course. The head was out but I didn't realise it. He gave me an injection into the vein and I was gone. When I woke up I wanted to go on with the birth. It was as though it hadn't happened.

For two months I cried. I went back at six weeks for my check-up to the gynaecologist. I was in floods of tears. He just opened the door and showed me out, patted me on the shoulder and told me I should keep busy. I went through various stages. I blamed the nurse. I blamed the doctor. I blamed myself. I felt nothing for the child. It took me a long time to feel anything for him. The birth was in May. From September to Christmas, I was on four different anti-depressants. I got three sessions of ECT [electro-convulsive therapy]. The psychiatrist said I would have no memory of the birth, and I thought that would be the best thing, to black it out of my mind. But it didn't work.

I used to go to this friar sometimes, just to talk to him. He said he couldn't be expected to understand postnatal depression, but he knew something about depression generally, the anger, the rage. My sister helped just by listening . . . There was a nun who was a healer. I used to go to the prayer group sometimes . . . It took me 15 months to get over it . . . So that was really why it took me so long to have another child and why I had the home birth.

❧

Moving Trolleys

'It's really a shining, sanitized cattlemart,' Lucinda says scathingly, speaking of the hospital environment. Her comment conveys some of the anger and resentment many women felt about their hospital births. Ulrike, from Germany, finds all the chrome and steel in hospital cold: 'It was so clinical, with tiled floors, hospital beds, plastic mattresses.' Such a view of the physical environment is widespread. It is sometimes difficult to know whether women are referring to qualities inherent in the materials – ceramic tiles are cold to the touch – or whether they are projecting on to the environment their feelings about their treatment at the hands of staff. Clearly, however, they are getting messages from the environment, ones that they do not like.

One aspect of the hospital's physical environment is the way it ensures, or fails to ensure, what women refer to as 'privacy'. When women talk about privacy, they are talking about who is around them, and about how appropriate it is, in their view, for that person to be there. 'The labour wards are horrible, very open and exposed,' Cora says. Sometimes, like Betty, women were talking about who could see them:

The screens were not pulled back properly, and another woman's husband saw the scissors-like thing they used to break my waters. I nearly died and he nearly fainted. It was very degrading.

This must be an example of what Kieran O'Driscoll, the Irish obstetrician, called 'mindless exposure in the indelicate lithotomy position'.[31] Women feel that multiple delivery units, containing up to four beds, separated only by curtains or screens, lack privacy. In such units, there is no feeling of intimacy, the intimacy that comes from having just one or two people in a room. No sense of enclosure, the enclosure that comes from having walls around you that do not move, and doors that need to be opened. And no feeling of security, the security of knowing that this is your space, that there is no possibility of seeing someone walk in without your permission. What women are complaining about, ultimately, is lack of control. 'It was like a public thoroughfare in there,' Efa says: 'Privacy is the main thing. Giving birth is very personal.' Open labour wards mean a lack of seclusion; they contribute to the feeling of being in a production unit. 'With all those pregnant women in the ward,' Frances says, 'it was like a conveyor belt.' Esther makes the hospital sound like a postal sorting office:

> They broke the waters at about seven. I was left there on a trolley. I was pushed from one place to another. All I could think was 'They're going to lose me'. They really were very busy. At one stage I was in the corridor. I was in somebody's way, and they just pushed me out of the way. At visiting-time, my husband came looking for me, and they couldn't find me.

Women object to the lack of exclusion. 'Even if you are a medical card-holder,' Máire says, remembering that she had no power to exclude anyone, 'you're lying there, and anyone can walk in, anyone.'[32]

Environmental factors may actually increase pain. In an open ward, fear of pain may be heightened by exposure at close range to the pain of others. Esther is crystal clear about how she was affected by the proximity of other women in labour:

> I was in with women in labour. There was a woman across the way, screaming in the labour ward. It was frightening to hear her. I remember one woman was in the height of labour, and I thought, 'Am I going to have to go through that?' Later I was in with women who had had miscarriages. There was one woman, her face was . . . [twisted]. I asked her what was the matter, and she said she was having a miscarriage. It was frightening.[33]

The absence of solid walls and single rooms means that there is always a sound factor, always the possibility of being exposed to the sound of other women and other births. Looked at in reverse, semi-public delivery units mean having to give birth as quietly as possible. This occasionally led to women being told to shut up by staff in the height of labour:

> If you made any sound at all, they would tell you to shut up, that you were disturbing the other patients [Mary].

Then there are the fittings for delivery, the furniture for birth. Particular censure is reserved for the standard hospital bed on which women are expected to deliver. Women complain that it is too high, that it is too narrow, and that it restricts their physical freedom:

> Even the bloody bed, there were steps up to it, so you had to climb on to it. Everything is geared to what suits them [Niamh].

There are the surfaces, the materials used for flooring, for example, which also came in for criticism. They have shining floors, Tríona says, but you feel you might slip on them if you want to get down off the trolley: 'It's not conducive to confidence.'

Even the hospital waiting-room is uncomfortable and unwelcoming, in Catherine's view:

> There's no comfortable place where a companion can wait for you. I've never known any place where you can make a cup of tea for someone, like you can, say, in a hotel room.

When the physical environment is badly designed, it has unintended consequences. In one hospital, if you were a public patient, whether or not you were separated from your baby depended on which postnatal ward you were allocated, as Geraldine, a former midwife in the hospital, explains:

If you were upstairs, the baby was taken away. They had a room for babies upstairs. If you were downstairs, the baby was left with you. They had no room for them downstairs.

Disinfectant in hospital is inevitable, but it triggers memories. Rachel, like others, finds the odour abhorrent; she refers to 'that whole, horrible, awful, clinical environment with that smell, the smell of Dettol'.

The physical environment always carries a message, as Patricia demonstrates:

We had to go into this small room to breast-feed, as if it was something filthy. It wasn't geared towards women's natural feelings.

᠅

Private and Public Patients

In Ireland, every woman is entitled to free maternity care in hospital. Some women pay for private care, for the privilege of having their 'own' obstetrician, of having their 'own' room after the baby is born. It makes them feel more cared for. They want to be more than a moving bump in a crowded clinic. They want to see the same face in labour that they have seen during pregnancy. Private care means consultant care, choosing an obstetrician for antenatal care who will then be legally responsible for your stay in hospital. In labour, whether you are a public or a private patient, you will be looked after by at least one midwife. The actual delivery – if uncomplicated – is also likely to be done by a midwife. And in most hospitals, public and private patients occupy the same labour and delivery units – private rooms are for postnatal use.

So who fares better, the public or the private patients? Women who have been public patients seem to think private patients do better, while those who have experienced private maternity care see advantages in going public. Florence (whose story appears on pages 31–2), equates being a public patient with meat processing. The treatment in hospital was ridiculous, she says, uncaring: 'You were just another body.' She denies the possibility that it might have been the staff on the day: 'It's their general attitude, particularly when you are a public patient.' Women who were public patients were more inclined to see maternity hospitals as baby factories, with normal labour as the assembly line, than women who were private patients.

But middle-class women who believe in natural childbirth often believe in the superiority of public care. 'I thought that public patients were better off. They had a better chance of a more natural delivery,' Frances, a former nurse, explains. She booked an obstetrician for her first baby: 'When the time came, he wasn't there.' Despite the fact that she wanted no 'interference', she ended up being induced: 'He wasn't ready to be born.' She was very angry about the birth, describing it as 'a nightmare'. She returned to the same obstetrician for the birth of her second child. Again, he was not there, and another doctor tried to remove the placenta: 'They just wanted to have everything over and done with by the time Dr Colbert came.' Obstetric care equals more intervention, women believe, a view which is borne out by some researchers.[34]

There are other discernible differences between public and private maternity care. Assumpta describes 'these two guys who came in and sat and watched [the birth]. When it was over, they went out again'. She is voicing a complaint that could only be made by a public patient. Private patients are not used routinely in the education of medical students. 'I had to delay the pushing until the doctor arrived,' Freda, a former midwife, observes. Again, she is expressing a grievance that could only be made by a private patient. Public patients are not delivered by named doctors.

In the last analysis, the decision to opt for public or private care – assuming that it is an option, financially – probably matters less than women believe. The fundamental complaints made by women about hospital maternity care, whether public or private, were identical.

Ultimately, bad hospital births were related, not to any individual shortfalls in standards of care, but to the structure and functioning of the system itself. In consultant-managed maternity units, birth *is* controlled by obstetrics.

Women want to be more than a component in what they see as the baby-processing industry.

3

Through the Looking-Glass

When you are having your first baby, you do not know anything. No matter how much you have read, you still do not know. The second time round, it is different. You can remember exactly. Largely because women could remember exactly, they decided to stay at home for the birth of this baby. They decided that instead of letting things happen, they would be in charge. This time, it was going to be different.

Home birth is an idea, to begin with. It is an idea that has never occurred to most women. It is not part of how we live any more. We have moved on, or so we think. 'They can do such wonderful things in hospital these days,' one woman was told by a doctor she met in the park, 'why don't you have your baby in hospital?'

In Ireland, there is virtually no alternative to the nearest high technology hospital. No happy medium, as some women see it. The hospital may be two hours drive away, but there is still no alternative. The alternative is to stay at home. Noelle had previously given birth at home, caught out by nature: 'Twice I hadn't been able to get there on time. It was a bit of a racket.'

How did women get the idea, that in this day and age, it was still possible to have a baby at home? The knowledge that, in Ireland, women of their own age had actually given birth at home, and lived to tell the tale, made a difference. Sometimes women stumbled across this knowledge in a letter to a newspaper. Or they happened to hear an interview on the radio, or they read an article in one of the women's magazines. Or somebody they knew had a home birth, and it went well. A friend could tip the balance, even at the eleventh hour. Angela always thought home birth was something hippies did, that it was irresponsible. She changed her mind after becoming pregnant:

> I thought I'd never go that far! It seemed to be a way-out thing to do. But a friend of mine had a home birth, and it was great. I got the names of a few midwives.

It is not a decision to be taken lightly. The support for the idea, socially, is nil, as the women in the group discovered. So what made them do it?

> I didn't like the thought of going to hospital, with all that poking and prodding, having no say in what happened. There is too much interference with the standard proce-dures, like induction, episiotomy, drugs. Telling me what position to adopt during delivery. I wanted my husband to be there. I wasn't sure that they would handle the baby gently afterwards, that he wouldn't be whipped off to a nursery. You have freedom when you are at home. The doctor and the midwife are guests in your house. They don't take over. You can have the children in immediately afterwards, then, later, you can all go to bed. As well as that, I had seen women lined up in the hospital waiting-room. It was very impersonal, they were all just numbers. I thought I would have an identity crisis if I went in there! [Emily]

Nearly all of the reasons why women have home birth are here. It is not a decision taken at random.[1] Being a patient means being powerless, having no control over what happens. Having to succumb to medical procedures you object to. Being told what to do. At home, it is a different equation, with professionals being referred to as 'guests'.[2] Guests do not take over, as Emily pointed out. In hospital, there is the added powerlessness of facelessness. Being a hospital patient may mean losing your 'self', having an identity crisis, as she said. At home, with your partner, and your children, if you have other children, around you, you never stop being yourself, women say. Finally, as Emily makes clear, birth doesn't stop with 'delivering' a baby. One minute you are pushing, the next minute the baby is out and you are watching others handle her. Having her handled gently, and not being separated from her, is something many women feel strongly about.

It is no wonder women find it so difficult to prioritize their reasons for having a home birth.[3] Their priorities interlock.

Many women detest being examined internally. 'I hated all that poking around,' Denise says. I had asked her why she decided to have Gerard at home, and not being poked around was the first thing that came to mind. Listening to women talk, they almost always recall some aspect of hospital practice or procedure that they object to. 'I just thought it would be nice to have a baby at home,' she continued. 'I wanted to be in my own bed, to do my own bits and pieces.' Being in control of labour is part of it, as always. There is also an element of curiosity: 'I wanted to see what it was like.' In common with other women in the group, Denise wanted to follow in her mother's footsteps: 'My mammy had the last three at home – she was 42 when she had her last – and I always wanted to do it, too.' Finally, home meant freedom from anxiety: 'I wanted to be able to take it easy at home.' For Denise, the birth represented an achievement, the fulfilment of an ambition frustrated for years, ever since the birth of her first baby in hospital: 'My experience on the first one really decided me to have Ashling (my second) at home.' But her doctor put her off. 'On Gerard [her third child], I suppose I got thicker [more stubborn],' she says. 'I decided I'd really look into it.'

A few women were having their 'last' baby. They saw this pregnancy as their only chance to have a home birth. Jo says she was very lucky:

I just happened to read a letter in the *Irish Times*, announcing a Home Birth Centre meeting. I knew it was going to be my last baby, so it was now or never.

Finally, two-fifths of the group had done it before. Repeat home births are common.[4] The decision to have your first home birth is the big one: mothers nearly always present subsequent home births as a foregone conclusion, like Linda:

Having had one at home, I couldn't imagine doing it in hospital. The hospital was fine as hospitals go, but I hated it. Birth is a fantastic experience.

POSITIVE POLES

༖

Taking Charge

I wanted to be able to enjoy the reproduction . . . to be free as a mother [Frances].

Psychologists talk about people's need to be in charge of their lives. Within the group, five out of every six women wanted to be in charge of their births. In countries where birth has been hospitalized, women's need for autonomy in this area of their lives is part of what is driving home birth.[5] Women see the home environment as their space, where the hospital hierarchy no longer applies. In your own house, women observe, you do not have to have anyone's permission to do anything. 'You can stand there stark naked if you want to,' Lelia says. Being free to do what feels right in labour, whether that means going for a walk or standing nude, is part of what women are seeking.

Two-thirds of the group believe in 'natural childbirth' (see Chapter 8). For them, being free to have a *natural* birth is what counts, as Penny explains: 'I didn't want the waters broken. I didn't want any drugs. I wanted to be allowed to follow my own instincts.' Women choosing home birth tend to believe in natural childbirth.⁶ It is only by remaining at home, they feel, that they will be free to produce this baby in their own time.

Many less well-off urban women believe pain medication in labour is unnecessary. They prefer to do without, if possible, to rely on themselves. Assumpta explains why she did not want pethidine. When she had it before, it dulled her senses: 'I wanted . . . to do it myself, with no interference.' 'It was not a natural childbirth thing,' she added. Some women want to do it for themselves. And for them, staying in control means doing without painkilling and anaesthetic drugs.

Wanting to have the experience is also part of why some women have home births and why they want to do without pain medication. According to Rosemary, in a clinical setting women are cheated of the emotional experience of giving birth. Motives can be tightly knit. If you want to have the experience, then wanting to have it 'in your full senses' – as many did – is the only thing that makes sense. If you see birth as significant, as most women did, being able to remember it matters. It is easier to remember it if you have not taken a drug such as pethidine. If you regard it as an experience, then you might well be curious, like Susan, a former nurse, 'to see what it would be like at home'. And if the event is so important, then you might want to ensure that it is by invitation only.

Wanting 'the privacy and aloneness' of a home birth, as Lucinda put it, represents the final strand of autonomy. Women see home as offering a cloistered place of their own, protected from public gaze, in which to labour and give birth. Privacy can only be ensured by restricting the view.

Birth is so important, women told me. How you see it is how it is. The more importance you attach to birth, the more necessary it becomes, not only to be able to experience it, but also to play a part in it. In hospital, women observe, it feels like other people have had the baby. Many women see home birth as an expression of their adult, female selves. It is a mark of independence, of a willingness to take responsibility.⁷ Lorna believes that you should not give over the most important experiences of your life, like birth and death, to a hospital. And Jean sees home birth in political terms: 'It links in with feminism, with being in control of my own body. I wish to take my own decisions.' Taking control, they feel, is also taking back something that obstetrics has taken away.

᠃

Knowing Your Midwife and Your Doctor

Within the group, women place enormous value on personal relationships. Birth is physical, they say, but the emotional side of it is more important. One of the features of a good birth, for many women, is one-to-one care from people that they know.

At home, Nuala says, you can build up a relationship with the nurse and the doctor. In hospital, smiles can become routine: 'They have probably delivered half a dozen babies that day already. There's no real value in sitting down and getting to know a patient.' Where antenatal care is provided by hospital antenatal staff, and care during labour is provided by labour ward staff, knowing your midwife is impossible. And where hospital midwives are not allowed to take private patients, choosing your midwife is impossible.

Denise felt she would be more relaxed at home: 'I would know the midwife, I wouldn't just be a piece of machinery passing through.' Not knowing your midwife, she implies, is tantamount to being processed by a machine operator. Assumpta says she wanted to know who was delivering her baby: 'I like being an individual. I wanted to be that person that it was all about, to be the centre of attention.' Some women felt that, at home, the standard of care was superior, that the level of attention was greater. Knowing your professional attendants means greater security. It means having a face, having a name. Feeling confident that you will have the support you need to get you through labour. Being able to ask questions more easily, and getting answers. Knowing that your feelings will be respected, your views listened to. It is the antithesis of depersonalized care.

ふ

A Family Affair

Birth is a family affair, a social thing, not a medical emergency [Rose].

In the Ireland of the 1940s, men had no role in childbirth. Unless, of course, they happened to be doctors. In Irish-speaking areas of Donegal, for example, the language of childbirth was known only to women. The Irish words and phrases used to describe labour and birth were passed from woman to woman. Men were excluded. Over the years, attitudes have changed. Natural childbirth has brought fathers into the birth chamber. Many women find their partners' presence helpful, to say the least. According to Noelle, it does something to the relationship, 'to be thrown this baby in a bath towel! He used to be terrified at the sight of blood!' Men's role in labour is part of what is driving home birth, worldwide.[8] In Ireland, an increasing number of fathers want to be involved. They feel that it improves their relationships both with their partners and with their new-born infants.[9] Within the group, three out of every four women wanted their partners to be present.

Romantic love could enter into the decision. Rachel was living in a rose-covered cottage down a hawthorn lane:

We'd bought this place. It was a dream. There was this aura about it. We fell in love with it. It was very romantic. It was our first home. I knew I wanted to have the baby in that room.

Being present is one thing, having a role is another. In hospital, Statia maintains, her husband would be a voyeur; at home, being able to go through labour without painkillers depends on his being there: 'It's either him or pethidine.' If women anticipate pain in labour, and natural childbirth is seen as a goal, then, like knowing your midwife, having your partner there may make all the difference.

Part of the impulse towards home birth is the conviction that birth is a family event, to be shared above all with your partner, and also with your other children, should you have them.[10] Involving children does not necessarily mean having them present at the actual birth. What many women wanted was to be able to call them in afterwards, when it was all over, when they felt ready for them. Many women feel that giving birth at home avoids the sibling jealousy and the jostling for attention that often accompanies the birth of a new baby.[11] There was no jealousy, Betty says, especially with the one who was the baby up until then: 'Their nose wasn't put out.' The bonding, they say, is better all round.

꩜

The Mother and Child Reunion

When you have a baby in hospital, it's their property [Irene].

I had these Leboyer ideas [Aylish].

It [the home birth] wasn't really for myself, but I didn't think the baby should be separated from the mother [Dympna].

Contrary to what must be inferred from what doctors have written,[12] women who choose home birth are deeply concerned about their babies. Many women wholeheartedly believe that home birth provides the best possible start in life for a baby. Martina says it was her belief that home birth was better for the child that gave her the strength to go through with her decision to have a home delivery: 'The nurse actually said to me "You want to kill your baby, don't you?"' Marilyn, having her second home birth, says the child was central to her decision:

[It was] the realization that a peaceful birth has a profound effect on the relationship that develops between mother and child, and on the subsequent personality of the human being. Birth is of the most profound importance in human relations.

Why do women feel the need to justify their decision in this way, when the issue is so multilayered? For Claire, as for others, it is simply part of being a 'good' mother: 'Making it easy for the baby to be born was the thing that made me decide in the end.' As the American writer Adrienne Rich shows, the 'good' mother is nurturing, selfless and self-sacrificing.[13]

When talking to women about what made them decide to have a home birth, names of writers such as Sheila Kitzinger or Frederick Leboyer often crop up. Grace says she read Leboyer's book, *Birth Without Violence*[14]: 'It said that glaring lights and loud noises were not good, and can hinder bonding.' She goes on to explain why the birth should be as relaxed and as welcoming for the baby as possible:

It's the baby's first impression of the world, so no smacks, noises or lights. These are their first thoughts. If the doctor mistreats them, they might get the idea that the world is not a friendly place, or that nobody loves them.

It is difficult to separate how women want their babies to be handled from how they see birth. Grace believes that birth affects the personality, that the child is imprinted indelibly by the experience of being born. As do others.

Women want to be able to handle their babies themselves, to bottle-feed on schedule or to breast-feed on demand, as they please. Home birth guarantees the cradle beside the bed, the baby in the bed, whatever you want. It is another reason for having a baby at home.[15]

NEGATIVE POLES

ༀ

Avoiding Procedures

At one level, home birth is an avoidance strategy. Three-quarters of the women in the group, as we have seen, had already had a baby in hospital. Many simply decided they were never going back. Dissatisfaction with and dislike of hospital is a large part of what is driving home birth.[16] It took her five years, Lucinda says, to have another child. She had a highly managed and deeply alienating first birth in a high technology hospital. It is partly because women object to how birth is managed in hospital that they feel they need more control over the process. Sometimes it was precisely because they had worked in a hospital that they felt this way. Emily had worked in a maternity hospital as a medical secretary. It left her with a terminal memory of what she saw as the 'attitude' of staff:

I don't like the way women are treated, the way they are abused . . . It was unbelievable, horrible. They were treated like lumps of meat.

Aylish was a midwife in the same hospital. She remembered births where, as she says, she would not like to have been the mother:

I saw that in hospital you had no control. Everything depended on who was on at the time. I felt I wouldn't be able to cope with labour as well as having to cope with difficult staff.

Home birth is as much a revolt against the obstetrical status quo as anything else.[17] Women do not like the exhortation to push during the second stage, or the rush to cut the umbilical cord before it has stopped pulsating, or any one of a number of practices routine in hospital.

Máire's memories are of enemas and episiotomies:

> Enemas are desperate things. I hate them. You're lying
> there with your legs wide open. God forgive me, but I felt
> like a cow hung up there. Enemas, episiotomies, the
> whole lot, it's degrading. I felt degraded. At home, you
> feel you're not being vandalized.

Remembered trauma creates all sorts of needs. Nuala says
Leesha's birth was the second reason why she stayed at home.
When the doctor was trying to break the waters, the baby was
not down far enough, she says, and it was very difficult. She
feels the birth was forced: 'They just bang you on to a drip.'
Being banged on to a drip is not what women want.

Over 40 per cent of women had taken pethidine, a drug
meant to dissociate you from the pain, on a previous labour.
For some, dissociation – feeling your head dislocated from
your body – was a distinctly unpleasant experience: 'The
pethidine had done me no good at all. I was up at the ceiling
looking down at myself, but I could still feel the pain.' Others
like Ellen object to the haziness, the loss of awareness, mind-
altering drugs induce:

> On my first, she was born at three and when my husband
> came in at eight, I was still completely drugged.
> Everything was very hazy. I was coming and going. I
> couldn't retain anything they said to me. It was terrible,
> on your first baby.

Side-effects such as loss of awareness and loss of control have
been widely reported in the literature.[18] For some women, the
loss of control they experienced was the worst feature of all.

Women occasionally feel that the pushing in hospital was
very forced: they bitterly resent being taken over in this way. A
'cattle station' Lucinda called the delivery suite. Angela says
her face was completely ruined when she was having Kean: 'I
had all these broken veins'.

Women felt strongly about not being on public display:

> With your two feet up in stirrups, you are in a very vulnerable position . . . There were six or seven midwives, a sister and a tutor. They were coming and going all the time.

There was no privacy, Deirdre concluded. What comes through is her sense of powerlessness, of having to deliver in a humiliating and demeaning position, in a space made public by virtue of the fact that unlimited and unknown staff can seemingly come and go at will. Having one's legs splayed apart in stirrups exacerbates the need for privacy. Being required to deliver a baby in this way is tantamount to being forced to have sex in public. Women found it indecent.

$\mathcal{S}$

Feeling Anxious

> When I found out I was pregnant, I was terrified of going into hospital [Florence].

The hospital would frighten the heart out of you, Máire says, recalling the big clock up on the wall: 'You'd be looking up at it and asking yourself, "How long more?"' Fear of hospital is common in women choosing home birth.[19] Given the 12-hour limit on labour, the clock is a perfect symbol of anxiety, a major factor, within the group, in two out of every three decisions. Asked what made her decide to have this baby at home, Kathleen replies: 'You know the way some people are afraid of heights? I'm afraid of hospitals.' Like a few other women, she has what doctors would call a 'phobia' about injections. But it was the induction of her fourth child that 'finished' her, she says, with hospitals. Her tenth child had come up in the sample for the study: it was her sixth home birth.

Losing control in hospital emerges again and again as a distinct thread in the fabric of women's anxiety. One of the ideas that natural childbirth has given women is the idea that they must control themselves in labour. Sue explains why she needed to avoid medical intervention:

> I had a fear of pain, and I didn't want to have to cope with intervention while in pain. I didn't want a shave or an enema. I felt that I would be able to cope if I was left alone. I dislike hospitals.

If you have a fear of hospital, in Cassie's opinion, you cannot control your labour: 'The state of your mind is very important. If you lose control, you're finished.' The link between fear, control and the environment is made by Aileen: 'I was afraid it [the birth] would be taken out of my hands. You can't make your own decisions out of your own environment.' The thought of not being able to refuse procedures that are in themselves painful is enough for Catherine, who recalls the horror of the drip, 'as if you weren't nervous enough already'. Women have a fear of being taken over. For many women, the loss of control that comes from being a patient is a major source of anxiety.

So is the anticipation of pain in labour. We are all awkward in pain, helpless, Harriet pointed out. For many women, labour is synonymous with pain. And this can lead to other anxieties of a very specific kind. Not everyone in the group believes in natural childbirth. Several women had not been able to get painkillers in hospital when they had asked for them during a previous labour. Being at home guaranteed access to pethidine, as far as they were concerned; their midwives carried pethidine. Being at home could also mean access to cigarettes. When you are a smoker, Betty observes, a cigarette relaxes you.

If there was no routine management of labour, no packaged delivery on offer, some women might have considered going to hospital. Statia says she would almost have a child in a field before she would have it in a hospital. Not every woman feels as strongly as this, but there is no doubt that the majority of women believe that staying at home is far less stressful than going to hospital. Women who believe in natural childbirth often worry about the possibility of doctor-induced damage in hospital. This anxiety is also part of what is driving home birth, worldwide.[20]

> I believe that the safest place to give birth is at home. It is not a medical event and treating it as such only leads to unnecessary complications [Ursula].

And they also believe that stress, in itself, can cause complications in labour.

⌁

The Threat of Separation

Patricia says she did not want to be away from her other two children:

> I was very close to them . . . If there was a facility to let the children be there, I might have gone in [to hospital]. As it was, it was bad enough trying to get them to allow your husband in.

She is not alone in this; the issue is raised by one woman in three. Enforced separation can be a source of acute anxiety for them, particularly when children are younger. They worry about how the children will react to their absence. They worry about who is going to take care of them, and how well. They see themselves as primarily responsible for their children's welfare. For some women, a stay in a maternity hospital is the only separation from their children they have known since they were born. For women who see themselves primarily as mothers, for women working full-time in the home, the prospect of even a short separation is extremely unwelcome.[21] What was in jeopardy, finally, was their view of themselves as mothers. Their identity was at risk.

Many women did not want to be separated from their husbands. Enforced separation from them during labour can be another source of anxiety.[22] For some women, a stay in another maternity hospital is the only separation from their husbands they have known since they got married.

They did not want to be separated from their newborn babies. As the American sociologist, Barbara Katz Rothman, has pointed out, the moment of birth is the ultimate separation of mother and child.[23] Rachel spoke about the coldness of the brass scales her baby was put into for weighing, after the warmth of where he had been. The scales were not even lined, she says. Not being separated again from your baby, just after you have brought her out into the world, is a topic raised by one woman in two.

The first days after birth, Thea observes, are very, very important: 'The babies should not be taken away and put into cots.' Just why those first days matter so much is rooted in research done by Marshall Klaus and John Kennell[24] who maintain that there is a critical period after birth, a time when the mother-child attachment can be permanently damaged if they are separated. Despite the lack of agreement on just what bonding or attachment is, many women have come to see the first hours, and days, after birth in this way.

৵

Comfort

What does comfort mean? Hospitals make me uptight. At home I can relax, and it's then easier to have a baby. My husband wanted to be at the birth and I liked having him there. I hate loads of people prodding and poking at me. The main reason was the comfort of home [Monica].

Lots of women talk about the *comfort* of home.[25] But do we know what they mean? I had asked Monica what she meant. Lack of anxiety is the first thing that came to mind. It is easier to give birth when you are relaxed, she points out. Hardly anyone would disagree with this. The importance of relaxation in labour is something that has been stressed for over sixty years, ever since Grantly Dick-Read wrote his book *Childbirth Without Fear*.[26] For Monica having her partner with her was part of it. To be reassured *is* comforting. It is also comforting to know that you do not have to undergo numerous internal examinations at the hands of strangers.

When women talk about comfort, they are often talking about freedom from anxiety. Harriet spells it out: 'Security, comfort. To be released from as much anxiety as possible.' For some women, freedom from anxiety is a prerequisite for an uncomplicated birth. Many women, like Ursula, see the outcome of labour as depending on one's state of mind. Again, she equates comfort with emotional security or freedom from anxiety:

> The safety of the baby and the comfort of the mother are totally interrelated. To be secure and relaxed in labour affects the labour. Where the spiritual and emotional aspects are given priority, they will determine the physical outcome.[27]

This is how women who believe in natural childbirth see it. In their view the well-being of the mother is synonymous with the well-being of the baby. Until the moment of birth, the two are one.[28] When doctors accuse women of selfishness, of putting their own comfort before the safety of the baby, this is what they fail to understand. Comfort has nothing to do with the physical ease of a deep armchair, a good bed or a luxurious bathroom. In the context of home birth, comfort means other things entirely, as Claire shows:

> The comfort of home is very important, both for the baby and for me. You're not upsetting the whole family. There's no big going away and coming back with a new baby.

Here it is as though comfort implies the security of unbroken continuous contact, with no threat of enforced separation. And there is the 'comfort' of knowing that the new baby will be accepted by the other children, without the jealousy women associate with the separation inherent in hospital birth.

Asked about how important the place of birth was to her, Hilda's reply reveals yet another dimension:

> It doesn't matter where it is so long as you are comfortable. You have to be totally at ease, as birth is an emotional experience. The people you choose are more important than the surroundings.

If she identifies comfort with being at ease, she also links it with the idea of knowing your midwife, with being able to choose your carers.

The last link in the chain is provided by Joan, who equates comfort with freedom from routine hospital procedures, such as repeated internal examinations:

> The comfort of staying at home, there's none of that pulling and poking. You're on your own ground. You don't have to put up with all that bull that you get in hospital.

And so we have come full circle. *Comfort* can be taken to mean any or all of the reasons for having a home birth, from freedom from anxiety and not being separated from your partner or from your other children, to knowing your carers and being on your own ground, or having some control. It is unsurprising that women talk about the comfort of home.

ᘒ

Charlotte's Story

Charlotte was having her fourth child at home; it was her second home birth. Her first birth in hospital she describes as 'undignified'. The staff were very busy. They could not find her folder. She was left in a corridor. They had no beds. Her husband was 'thrown out'. When he went back in later, he says, 'She'd had nothing to eat. She was left for hours without attention.' Charlotte takes up the story:

> I had backache. There was one midwife who rubbed my back and told me I was going to be all right. That was the only humane part of the whole thing. On a first baby, you don't know whether you're going to be able to produce that baby or not. There was no reassurance.

Afterwards she was sick, vomiting from the effects of the gas she had been given. Her baby was taken away, and put into an incubator because she was 'small' (see pages 41–2).

When Charlotte found herself pregnant again, she tried to organize a home birth: 'I didn't want Rachel [who was fifteen months old at the time] to go to her granny's. It was enough for me to be leaving the house.' A fruitless search for a midwife followed. She was forced to return to the hospital, stayed for five days, and came home to find Rachel had forgotten her.

Her mother had had four children at home, but it was her sister who influenced her, she says. She had had a home birth before Charlotte. She wanted to have some say over what happened to her: 'In hospital you don't assert yourself . . . You have more control over the situation at home.' She continues:

> From the children's point of view, you're not away. I suppose I'm a bit of a mother hen! . . . It's a family thing, birth. In hospital you're separated from your husband, although that's beginning to change. It's his baby too.

Then there was 'the lack of a personal touch', and, finally:

> This injection they wanted to give me . . . I thought, 'Why can't I produce a baby naturally?' I wouldn't take drugs from the child's point of view. If I did, I'd feel lousy about

it afterwards . . . I wanted something natural, not making it into an operation with drugs.

She says she is not a 'hospital person':

As a child I spent five years in hospital . . . My sister died when I was fourteen. My brother, my sister, and myself were taken into hospital for tuberculosis. I got spinal meningitis. They said later I'd probably picked it up in there. I was four and a half years old when I went in.

Alienated by her childhood experiences, Charlotte has moved away completely from orthodox medicine: 'No aspirins, no antibiotics, no vaccinations . . . I'd rather cope with the illness than cope with the side-effects of the vaccine.' She and her family now attend a naturopath two hundred miles from where they live.

It was a joint interview. Charlotte and her partner appeared to be a very united couple. He had the last word: 'I delivered him . . . Birth is not exclusive to mothers.'

UNDER THE INFLUENCE

☙

Men

It is difficult to know what influence a man has on his partner's decision to have a home birth. Many women are quick to point out that, ultimately, they carry the can for this particular one. According to a Dutch psychologist, Gunilla Kleiverda, women tend to make this decision themselves,[29] and this was borne out within the group.

Middle-class women tend to emphasize how important it is to have a supportive partner. Lesley says she could not have contemplated a home birth without good, caring, loving support from her husband. When a woman who is pregnant announces that she wants to have this baby at home, the response can sometimes be less than enthusiastic. Less well-off women are not always convinced of the need for their partners' approval, let alone co-operation. They regard the decision as theirs, and theirs alone. A small number of women actually went ahead with their plans despite sustained opposition from their husbands. What Denise recounts is typical: 'In the beginning, he wasn't very keen, but he came around, once he realized I was having it at home whether he liked it or not.' Middle-class women, many of them feminists, would not have dreamt of taking this kind of line. In middle-class families, sharing is the norm,[30] making unilateral action less likely.

In a minority of cases, men played a central role in the decision-making process. Nine per cent of fathers took part in the study uninvited: some of them were outraged that the research project was confined to women.

꒰

In Your Mother's Footsteps

After, or indeed sometimes before your partner, there is your mother to consider. And your father. Women were influenced, sometimes strongly, by what their mothers said or did. Like several others in the group, Dympna's mother was a midwife: 'She did home deliveries 25 years ago – the last one was in 1965. I was born at home.' In giving birth at home, nearly half of the group were following in their mothers' footsteps. Geraldine sums up the general effect of this: 'My mother had had two of us at home, so it was something that could be done.' These women felt that it was safe in some way, that it was normal. In every second case, women – mostly less well-off, urban women – made it clear that following in their mothers' footsteps was something they were consciously aware of. Nuala says her main reason for having a home birth was the fact that her mum had her at home. Nuala's mother did not actually plan on having her at home, and she haemorrhaged afterwards, but it made no difference to Nuala: 'I always wanted to do it.'

Fathers' influence on their daughters was less obvious. Nine women brought up the fact that their fathers were doctors. I did not ask. In Virginia's case at least, it must have made a difference. Her father was a general practitioner in the south of England, and he specialized in home deliveries.

Women were more likely to be influenced by their sisters than by their sisters-in-law. Jean's sister had had a baby at home three years before: 'I wasn't at the birth, but I was in the house. It impressed me a lot.' Several women were influenced by female members of their own family, but none seemed to attach any importance to home births on their husband's side of the family.

Not all mothers were favourably disposed to the idea of their daughters having a home birth. They did not necessarily want a home delivery for their daughters just because they had had one themselves. Kathleen, who was having her tenth child, continued to live at home after she got married:

> For the first four I was living in me mother's. She wouldn't hear of it. She just didn't want the responsibility. It wasn't until we got this house that I could stay at home.

With every addition to the family, you move up on the public housing list. Whilst Kathleen had to wait until she got a house of her own, four children later, before she could have a home birth, Rita had to wait even longer. Her first two children were born in hospital:

> My mother made me because I had Rhesus Negative blood . . . After my mother died, all the rest of my babies were born at home.

༈

Memory

I remember when home birth was perfectly normal, a street event. Neighbours would bring in soup, take away the washing [Fionnuala].

Being able to remember the birth of a sister or brother at home is reassuring. Like knowing a friend who had a home birth, it makes the idea of doing it yourself more real. Memories of babies born at home locally have the same effect. Mary recalls the changing times in the early 1950s:

I was born at home, the youngest of a big family. All of us were born at home. The nurse lived at the end of the road. The younger mothers were going into hospital to have their babies, but the older ones were still having them at home. I grew up thinking it was normal.

It is hard for us to imagine how normal home delivery was in those days. As a tradition, it lingered on: in Dublin the major maternity hospitals operated a district service until the 1960s. Mona recalls the district midwives: 'They looked great, in their blue uniforms and their bicycles.' Such memories are powerful. Listening to less well-off, urban women, the impression gained is that childbirth had not yet been taken over by obstetrics. They still saw birth as an everyday part of life.

For the majority in the group, hospital birth is the norm. They did not have memories of district midwives. But for women who came to live in Ireland, it could be a different story. In England, Jane says, you were expected to have your second child at home. Writing in the *British Medical Journal*, an English general practitioner, Dr Shearer, recalls that in 1954 only women with problems and a few first-time mothers were able to book a bed for delivery in the local hospital.[31]

In the Netherlands, as late as 1960, home births accounted for three-quarters of all births.[32] Over the last fifteen years, they have levelled off, nationally, at around 35 per cent.[33] For Beatrix, the decision to have a home birth was a foregone conclusion:

> I never considered anything else. If you are from Holland, it is different. It was later I realized how difficult the choice was here [in Ireland].

When home birth is part of the way people live, then it can be seen as part of the culture of a community or a country. In the case of women like Beatrix born outside Ireland who see themselves as alternatives, there is a coming together of two cultures. Home birth since the 1960s has been seen as part of the 'alternative health' movement,[34] part of the 'hippie' lifestyle, or what is called 'the counterculture'. If home birth is part of her national culture for Beatrix, it is also part of the way she lives now. Comparing the Irish system of maternity care where home birth is on the periphery, to the Dutch where it is at the centre, she comments that in Ireland: 'It was the other way around!'

For Beatrix, and other alternatives, it is also the other way around. If you live on the edge of society, then the decision becomes whether or not to come into the centre. Sometimes it is just too difficult. And if you live deep in the heart of nature, the nearest large-scale, high-technology hospital is just too far away.

Women who decide to have a home birth want to take childbirth back into their own hands. They have ideas about natural birth or wanting a 'gentle' birth for the baby. To put these and other ideas into practice, they feel they need to be able to call the shots.

Women have emotional needs in birth. They want to be looked after in labour by people they know. They want to be talked to, to be looked at, to be listened to, when they are having a baby. They want privacy and intimacy in birth. They want to share it with the family. They want their partners to be there, their other children to be around.

Having just pushed this baby out into the world, they do not want to be separated from her. Women who had experienced home birth talked about bonding with the new baby, about avoiding jealousy among the older ones. Curiosity can be a motive. Some women always wanted to have a baby at home. Some wanted to see what it would be like. Because their mothers had done it, some wanted to do it too.

Some could remember neighbours having babies at home. It did not seem abnormal. Sometimes a close friend had had a home birth, sometimes a sister. It did not seem dangerous. For women living an alternative lifestyle, home birth is almost normal. And for women from the Netherlands, it is completely normal.

In countries where it is not normal, home birth is a revolt by women against the way obstetricians manage birth in hospital. If home birth is about giving fathers a role, it is because it is only at home that women can be sure he will be there. If it is about avoiding intervention, it is because only at home can women be certain that medical procedures will not be forced on them. It is because only at home can women be sure they will be listened to.

Women fear hospital. They have nightmares about being out of control, about being looked after by unknown midwives on shift. For nearly every woman, home birth is an avoidance strategy, and women who believe in natural childbirth have more to fear than those who do not. Two-thirds of the group believe that the drugs, instruments and machines routinely used in hospital carry substantial risks.

For all of these women, going out on a limb made sense.

ॐ 4 ॐ

Stone Mad

They all thought I was stone mad, family, friends, neighbours. My colleagues told me I should know better. My obstetrician was completely against it [Freda, a former midwife, currently nursing].

Of all the problems women may encounter during pregnancy, locating a midwife is not usually one of them. If you are having a baby in hospital, you do not even have to think about the service. It is just there. For women planning a home birth in Ireland, nothing is in place. In a country where nearly every woman has her baby in hospital, locating professional help can be a huge problem. In rural areas, finding a midwife is like looking for a needle in a haystack. The number of independent midwives – certified nurse-midwives – in private practice does not amount to more than a dozen altogether. There were about half a dozen general practitioners in the country, three of them in Dublin, as well as one obstetrician, taking maternity cases. For most women, persuading their doctor to do it, usually against his will, was their only chance. Most midwives were reluctant to work without medical cover.

For some women, the months of pregnancy were fraught with doubt and uncertainty, with the planned home birth in jeopardy until the very end. It was a time of conflict – doing battle with hostile doctors or aggressive health officials. Women were constantly being told by everyone that they were putting two lives on the line, not *just* their own, but their baby's. The pressure to have this baby in hospital was enormous. Nine months is a long time.

If home birth means having the baby yourself, it also means doing all the work yourself. And as often as not, doing it on your own. In households where preparations were made for the birth, half of the fathers involved themselves in such activities as reading; the other half did not.

Women talked about having to know more at home, so they could have their arguments ready. Many read whatever they could find on the topic. Some joined one of the birth organizations. Knowing someone else who had had a home birth made them feel less deviant.

Doctors who accuse women wanting a home birth of not caring about their babies would be hard put to explain the care and attention these women lavished on themselves in pregnancy,[1] watching what they ate, what they drank, doing exercises. And if they did not always have the recommended amount of antenatal care, it was often because they got tired of being harrassed or intimidated over their decision. Or because they were afraid of being shipped into hospital.

～

Planning This Pregnancy

'Smear test results showing abnormal cells precipitated the decision to have this baby then,' Martina says, recalling her anxiety about cervical cancer. She was in a minority. Just 42 per cent of babies were planned. About the same number were conceived by chance – Claire's was a 'progesterone only' pill baby – and the rest were neither planned nor unplanned. In a country where women's control over their fertility has traditionally been limited, having an unplanned baby is not too difficult. And several women made it clear that they preferred to use 'natural' as opposed to 'artificial' methods of contraception.

ℜ

Finding a Midwife

Women in Ireland are legally entitled to a maternity service at home.[2] Applying to the state for information about a state service makes sense. Rose, a nurse, describes how they made her feel deviant in her local health clinic the first time she went to them:

> They told me to go and discuss it with my GP. They said the midwives weren't experienced . . . You could sense their fear.

Deborah, a former nurse, pinpoints one possible reason for anxiety among health board staff: 'I heard that the superintendent public health nurse asked later was I the type to sue.' Hilary also went to her local health board. She was told she was being selfish in wanting a home birth:

> They told us it was unsafe. That their midwives were not trained to do home births. That they didn't have anybody. So we put an ad in the papers, and we got six responses.

Only a very small number of women managed to get a midwife through their local health board. Sometimes it was actually one of the board's own employees, a sympathetic public health nurse, who agreed to do the delivery. There was nobody doing home births, health boards told women, over and over again. But there were midwives out there, somewhere, who were willing to do it, as women who advertized in newspapers found out.

There are easier ways of finding a midwife than going to your local health clinic. Contacting one of the birth organizations, such as the Home Birth Centre, is one of them. A quarter of the group found their midwives through the birth 'underground'. Once they got into the network, Aileen says, arranging the birth was easy. But not everyone was part of the network. Living in one of the poorer urban districts, or in a rural area, made it more difficult.

Even in a small country where so much depends on who you know, finding an experienced community midwife could be a major headache. 'All I knew was that her name began with an E,' Dympna says, referring to her midwife. She had a friend doing a university course in co-operatives, the lecturer's wife had had a home birth, and she told her there was a midwife in a particular county. Dympna and her husband moved house. And Charlotte, pregnant with her fourth child and living in a rural area, ran it to the wire. She had spent years looking for a midwife. One week before this baby was due, an independent midwife arrived home from New Zealand, and Charlotte booked her.

Irish midwives in private practice work on their own, without the kind of cover a group practice would provide. Netta was praying that when she went into labour, a number of other women would not follow suit. Her midwife was only fitting her in as a favour: 'She had a few booked around the same time as me.' Multiple bookings could make for sleepless nights.

A fifth of the group simply contacted their former midwife – from a previous home birth. But having a repeat home birth does not guarantee a midwife. Dora's former midwife had died. She persuaded her family doctor to do it, and arranged for her local public health nurse to come in afterwards. Arrangements were makeshift sometimes. They had to be.

Making a backdoor arrangement was not unknown, either. Sinéad persuaded a friend, who was a hospital midwife, to deliver her baby. Pat's midwife was a nurse who had done her midwifery: 'The doctor who was my GP suggested her. It was a personal favour.'

ぅ

Talking to Doctors

Most midwives did not work without medical back-up. So if you wanted a home birth, you had to find a family doctor who would agree to be on standby when the time came. This was easier said than done.

Women in the group reported how the names of doctors known to do home births could be got from one of the birth organizations. Outside the underground, professional referral was the second most common way of getting help, with community midwives giving women the names of doctors who did home deliveries, and vice versa. Personal contact was the third. Everything, in a way, depended on knowing someone.

If you did not know anyone, it could be hard to know where to begin. You might make the mistake Rachel made in going to her local doctor: 'She was very nervous, hospital-oriented.' 'Why risk this baby's life?' she asked her. Rachel then tried another doctor in the area, who also refused. Hit-and-miss surgery consultations like this could be fruitless, and upsetting.

Most women wanted a general practitioner to be on call for the birth. Frances went to her GP, and asked him what did he think of home births: 'He said he didn't think of them.' That was the end of that. A fifth of the group managed to persuade their family doctor to be in attendance. Sometimes, persuasion was a long drawn-out process, more like a war of attrition: 'One week the doctor would say he'd do it, and another week, he'd say he wouldn't,' Sinéad says.

It could be the luck of the draw. Several elderly doctors saw this delivery as a final achievement before they retired. Claire, a nurse, says her GP was very helpful once he realized she was taking an 'intelligent' approach. For those lucky enough to live in a city or town where a local general practitioner or obstetrician was known to do home births, it was easy. The only other possibility was to seek out whoever had attended your mother in childbirth; within the group, there were eight second generation deliveries.

⤳

Beatrix's Story

The local doctor upset me very much. He was full of horror stories. Then I found an old nurse: she was lovely. It was a back-door agreement. She would come if I called her in the middle of my labour, but it was not official. If she did it officially, she would lose her job.

Beatrix and her partner moved to another part of the country, and she had to begin all over again. By then, she was nearly eight months pregnant:

I got on my bike and went to all the doctors in the area. There were five or six of them. There was one doctor left. He was in his late fifties: he had done a lot of home deliveries when he was younger. He let me talk about why I wanted a home birth.

The doctor agreed to do it. There was only one difficulty – he wanted a midwife to be in attendance:

I was told there was no midwives in the area. I knew the local community nurse didn't really want to do it. You can't force people. She kept on trying to dissuade me right up to the end. She was very Catholic. She said she would pray for me. I told the doctor she didn't really want to do the delivery, and in the end, he accepted.

In the end, the doctor's wife acted as a substitute midwife. The doctor had not done a delivery for 25 years.

᠎ౢ

A Public Service

Eileen applied to her local health board for a maternity service: 'They said, "You can't have it" . . . There was a clamp-down at that time.' Angry parents have more than once resorted to the law in an attempt to compel the state to provide them with a midwife or a doctor at home. The 'clamp-down' was the board's response to a legal action brought against it by frustrated parents attempting to force the board to carry out its obligations under the 1970 Health Act.[3]

This is the background against which the state provides a home birth service, such as it is. Contracted out to individual midwives and doctors, the state pays and women make their own arrangements with the professionals involved. How they find them in the first instance is another day's work. Information-giving is the first arm of the service, and health boards carry information on community midwives, but not on general practitioners willing to accept maternity patients.

Half of the women who contacted their local health board were discouraged from going ahead with their plans. Sometimes, of course, what women saw as discouragement could be unintentional. If the board sent out information on midwives who turned out to be either dead or retired, women usually took this badly. It did not occur to them that it could be just lack of interest, or knowledge, or both, on the part of staff. There were times when discouragement could be unambiguous, however. To say that Statia was discouraged would be an understatement:

> I was asked had I any consideration for the child. It was no good trying to explain that it was precisely because I had consideration for the child that I wanted a home birth.

Sometimes the pressure bordered on bullying. Again and

again, the threat of mortal danger is emphasized: 'The super-intendent public health nurse said I was risking two lives,' Susan said, 'not just my own, but the baby's.'

Getting a service from the state can be problematic for other reasons. Some women have no idea of what they are entitled to.[4] This is a feature of health and welfare services everywhere. When you read the forms you understand why. Less well-off women tend to be less well informed about their entitlements. The state does not have to advertize its services in this area. If you do not know about it, you cannot apply for it.

Sometimes the service worked as it should. Two-thirds of the group persisted with their application for midwifery or medical services. Outside Dublin, more often than not, the service was provided through clenched teeth, as Penny shows:

> When I first wrote to them, they sent me a letter saying that according to all the obstetricians, hospital was the only safe place in which to give birth, that I was behaving irresponsibly in wanting to have a home birth and that there were no facilities for home births. I wrote back and said that I was going to have my baby at home and that I wanted a midwife. They gave me the names of two midwives. One of them was no longer doing it, and the other was old, and had no transport.
>
> I wrote again and said I was going to have my baby at home, that I had my GP. So two weeks before the birth, the nurse came out to ask me if I was still going to have a home birth, and I said I was. And the following day, they got me a midwife. She lived only a few miles from here.

Exactly the same kind of brinkmanship can be seen in Tríona's case. Again, the health board took no action for months, but she persisted with her request for a service. Then, five days before her baby was due, a local doctor was conscripted by the board and a volunteer midwife recruited from the local hospital. Any health board wishing to thwart a pregnant woman's plans for a home birth only had to stall her until her deliver-by date was past, to ensure a hospital delivery – or an unattended birth. Two women who tried and failed to get a midwife from the state went on to have a non-attended birth (see Chapter 7).

Technically, only 12 per cent of women who looked for a midwife failed to get one. However, a number of women who were eligible for the service did not even apply. They had got their fingers burnt on a previous occasion.

In the south of the country, the position of community midwifery was fragile. The regional health board felt itself to be under siege, caught between the prongs of an ever-increasing demand for home birth in a region where alternative life-styles were common, the conviction that home births were dangerous, and fear of litigation.

Virginia lived in the war zone. Her midwife had trained in England:

She was doing home deliveries in a private capacity while working in the local hospital. The board told her they wouldn't ratify her Irish qualifications, if she carried on doing home deliveries. Mine was the last she did.

The conflict between women and the board was fought on various fronts, on sites which ranged from health clinics to private homes and local hospitals. Mary's midwife was barred from the local hospital:

She couldn't even get the injection that they need for the Rhesus. She wanted to get an oxygen thing for the baby. She couldn't even get that either.[5]

In failing to provide a maternity service to women at home, health boards are in breach of their statutory obligations. But what does the service amount to? Linda describes how it worked for her: 'They sent me a form, and said that I would be liable for anything over £30 myself.' The statutory fee paid to midwives worked out at around £1 an hour, depending on the length of labour: the fee covered up to five antenatal and not less than ten postnatal visits. To add insult to injury, the usual travel and subsistence allowances payable in the public service were not as a rule paid to independent midwives in rural areas.

Nuala, an unsupported mother with three children, dependent on social welfare, found herself caught between the official fiction that the delivery could be done for £30 and the reality:

> I had booked the midwife. I got on to the Eastern Health Board about the maternity pack. I said, 'What's £85 for an experience that you want?' She said, 'You shouldn't be charged anything. You don't pay when an Eastern Health Board nurse does it.'

One week later, Nuala got a letter from the midwife she had booked telling her she could not do the delivery, and referring her to a midwife in private practice. This midwife charged Nuala a fee of £120, which showed that the original 'top-up' fee of £85 was almost exactly the difference between the state fee and the private fees being charged at the time. Top-up payments were the norm. If you want to have a home birth, women remark, you have got to have the money.

᠀

Antenatal Care

Antenatal care has been defined as a system 'whereby pregnant women attend for medical examinations and testing at the pre-set intervals of monthly to 28 weeks, fortnightly to 36 weeks, and weekly thereafter'.[6] Although they were in a minority, a number of women did not have the recommended amount of antenatal care. A third of the group did not see a doctor or a midwife until after the fourth month of pregnancy, and half of these women put off going to see a doctor until they were six months pregnant or more. A tendency to under-utilize systems of antenatal care among women planning a home birth has come up in other studies.[7] Pat said the gynae was 'singularly unpleasant' to her:

88

He said it [having a home birth] was irresponsible, and he hoped the hospital wouldn't have to take responsibility if anything went wrong.

The possibility that the hospital will be liable if anything goes wrong is a recurring theme. One visit to a hospital antenatal clinic, and you are 'their' patient for the duration of your pregnancy and birth. Obstetricians, like hospitals and health boards, are afraid of being sued.

The discouragement women having a home birth experience from GPs, from hospital midwives, and from health board staff has a knock-on effect, and the effect is negative. Mary Ellen describes how she used to come out in tears from the hospital antenatal clinic:

There were two midwives, who headed the midwives' clinic, who ate me every time I went. Psychologically it wore me down, all these horror stories. They said I wasn't a suitable candidate for home birth, because of 'my poor muscle tone', because it was 'my fourth baby', and because of 'my age' [thirty-one].

Medical hostility to home birth only drives women deeper underground. In Canada, doctors' refusal to give antenatal care to women planning a home birth led, not to more hospital births, but to less antenatal care.[8]

There are other reasons why women do not avail themselves of antenatal care in the recommended amounts. They may have lost faith in orthodox medicine. They may not believe pregnancy is a disease. They may feel antenatal care is hyped up to be so much, and then it takes all of three minutes, in and out of the surgery or the clinic, after waiting for three hours.

Half of the group were looked after during pregnancy by general practitioners, with half as many again supplementing GP care with hospital, obstetrician or midwife care. Traditionally, family doctors provided women with routine antenatal care and midwives looked after women during labour, calling a doctor only in the event of complications. Three women in the group got sole care from a midwife. As many as 15 per cent of women attended an obstetrician privately, often augmented by GP or midwife care. Not everyone in obstetrics shares the view that home births are inherently dangerous.

Routine antenatal surveillance hinges on blood, urine and blood pressure testing. A quarter of the group had ultrasound. By hospital standards, this was very low. But for women getting their antenatal care in the community, scanning is not routine, and within the group, health problems were few. Some women had ultrasound for suspected twins, or because their delivery dates were uncertain. Sometimes ultrasound seemed like an insurance policy, with home birth seen as an additional loading on the premium. Several GPs ordered scans 'just in case'. Not every woman wanted a scan: there was a growing view that ultrasound scanning could carry un-dreamed-of risks for the baby. No one had an amniocentesis, although a fifth of the group were aged 35 or over: an ante-natal test to detect genetic and chromosome problems in the fetus, it is not widely available in the Irish Republic.

When you are pregnant, doctors tell you to take iron and vitamins. Only half of the group took this advice. Cecilia did not take iron tablets because 'there was a suggestion that iron was related to jaundice'. Others defined iron as medication, and refused to take it. Women generally avoided medication in pregnancy like the plague. A quarter of the group took no pills of any kind.

Like a small number of women, Pat prefers to take homeo-pathic medicine:

> Homeopathic iron from nettles. Rose iron. Homeopathic calcium that enhances your body's ability to produce calcium. Caulophylum to give you an easier labour. Lime blossom baths to expand the cervical area. Arnica D6 for any kind of disturbance, to put the body into harmony before, during and after labour.

Caulophyllum and raspberry leaf tea, both believed by some women to tone the womb, were favourites in pregnancy.

࿂

Parsley, Seaweed and a Glass of Stout

As a biology teacher, Sian believes that pregnancy, not birth, is the vital time for the baby: 'That means adequate nutrition, no smoking, no alcohol.' Women choosing home birth are known to be especially concerned with what they eat.[9] Ruth, like two-thirds of the group, believes her diet to be healthy: 'I'm very aware of food. I go in for wholefoods, a little meat, free-range eggs and homemade bread.' Others, describing their diet as 'normal' or 'mixed', say they pay no special attention to what they eat.

Having a *healthy* diet could mean anything from avoiding junk food to being a vegan or a macrobiotic. The stereotype of home birth mothers as vegetarians has a grain of truth: within the group, one woman in every five was a vegetarian, which is double the national average in Britain, for example.[10] However, hardly anyone was on a macrobiotic or a vegan diet.

During pregnancy, a third of the group made specific improvements to what they regarded as a good diet. These women tended to eat more fruit, raw vegetables and leafy greens. Some of the women were stringent about what they ate and drank, cutting out tea or coffee, or both, to ensure a healthy pregnancy. A small number of women did not drink tea or coffee anyway, ever. Improvements to diet are a matter of opinion: some women cut out dairy products, for example, while others increased them. Meat-eaters ate more liver.

Several women mentioned eating things like apricots, or parsley. Pregnant women and nursing mothers used to be encouraged by their doctors to drink a glass of stout. A few women drank a glass of Guinness regularly, while others took cod liver oil, a less pleasant tonic. Supplementing your diet with calcium (recommended by some midwives),[11] yeast extract, seaweed and vitamin E was something some women did, but it was not usual.

Of the 49 per cent who drank alcohol, a third cut back or cut it out completely during this time. Others reported that it had lost its taste. Of the 44 per cent of women who smoked – mostly the kind the government taxes – half reduced the habit or gave it up during pregnancy. Philomena, who was having her eighth child, explains why she reverted to smoking during this pregnancy:

> The sixth took an hour, but he was 12 lbs 3 oz! I gave up smoking during the last month, and I put it down to that.

She continued to smoke during her first five pregnancies. Up until then, she explained, her babies had all been a normal weight, and her labours were always short.

꙳

Toning Up

Philomena continued to go to local dances with her husband during her pregnancy. Nearly half of the group did specific exercises for pregnancy and birth, regularly, and most women put on between 12 and 35 lbs during this time. Women who did not exercise in this way were often run off their feet already. Asked about exercises for pregnancy and childbirth, Harriet says she had lots of laundry to do: 'We had no running water, so I had enough exercise, I thought, even if it wasn't the right kind.' Women with small children to look after, as she did, often felt they were just too busy looking after them to do anything else.

Within the group, women preferred to do traditional exercises, such as breathing and relaxation exercises, rather than things like pelvic floor exercises or squatting. Walking was a favourite. A few continued to swim, or to do yoga, while others preferred cycling, jogging or running. Leslie continued to go horse-riding, and she also kept up her dance classes. A small number of women did perineal massage, which involved opening up the birth canal, gradually, with the hand, to prepare it for the width of the baby's head.

༄

Eye Contact and Block Appointments

Having one's preferences taken into account was a feature of antenatal care women valued. Catherine was very pleased with her doctor: 'You're the only patient I've ever examined from the other side of the room,' he told her once. (She had put internal examinations off-limits.) Two out of every three women getting their antenatal care from a general practitioner were very satisfied. For the most part, women tend to single out the doctor's clinical skills, although being made to feel at ease by their doctor is something less well-off women bring up.

Maeve, a nurse, says she had every confidence in her midwife:

> She seemed to be very intuitive. I was very relaxed with her. She was clinical in her thoroughness, yet she was a friend. There was a feeling that you were in it together.

The few women who were looked after during pregnancy by an independent midwife were very pleased with their care. However, the traditional way of doing things meant that some women experienced care as fragmented. If they saw a doctor in pregnancy, that doctor was often only on standby for the birth. It also meant that some women had little or no contact with their midwives before going into labour. There were occasional complaints about midwives being strangers.

Rachel, a nurse, thought her antenatal care, both from her GP and from the hospital, very poor:

> If they gave out the sticks, you could test your urine at home. If you look after yourself, if you are educated, there isn't any need for all this running to the doctor. Antenatal care is hyped up to be so much, and then it amounts to very little . . . They don't even look at you.

When asked about antenatal care, women frequently mention aspects of communication which they find unsatisfactory.[12] Statia says doctors are 'non-communicative': 'There's no eye contact. They're looking down at your feet, and saying, "Have you felt any movement?" '

Public antenatal clinics are the targets for harsh criticism. Carole was disgusted by the block appointments system: 'The queue. Forty women waiting on the bare boards. No appointments. Everyone told to come at two o'clock.'[13] Rachel describes women being lined up on benches with their bumps, 'like cattle'. Block appointments inevitably mean queues. Being forced to sit around for hours, wearing a hospital gown, waiting to be called in for examination, is bad enough, women feel. The way Katherina described the hospital, it sounded more like an animal testing station than a women's antenatal clinic:

> I was appalled at the mass check-ups. Five of us were told to go in, take off our clothes and lie on the beds. Then they pulled the curtains and the doctors came around.

It is difficult to know how widespread this particular system of antenatal surveillance was. Maybe this was the only one of its kind. But Katherina was not the only woman to feel degraded by the experience. Tríona singles out a standard feature of public clinics:

> It was inhuman, like cattle at the mart. The compartmentalization, one midwife takes the blood pressure, another does something else. There is no continuity.[14]

Depersonalized care strips women of their dignity. Just as a woman's satisfaction with antenatal care could indicate a good relationship with the professional involved, such dissatisfaction with public clinics within the group could also, however, reflect a poor view, overall, of maternity hospitals.

ॐ

'You're Very Brave'

Everyone thought I was cracked. But I am very calm. I
don't get bothered [Dora].

Independent midwife, Caroline Flint, says that of the minority
of women who want home births, only the most determined
actually succeed.[15] There is no record of those who do not, but
hostility from health professionals *is* well documented.[16] Being
warned by professionals is one thing however; being dissuaded
by your husband or your mother is another. Florence says her
husband was against it: 'It didn't bother me. I felt it was I who
was having the baby.' Like Florence, seven women in the group
had to contend with opposition from their partners right up to
the bitter end. None of them seemed unduly put out by it.

Angela's mother was very upset, initially. After a few weeks,
she changed her views: 'I was expecting much more resistance,' Angela commented. Her mother had discussed the
matter with her family doctor, a medical practitioner of the old
school, who was still doing home births. Niamh's father was
totally against the idea, too. If he thought it was safe, she says,
he would not have minded. It seemed as though there was no
end to the disapproval:

The neighbours thought I was off the rails. They said
you'd have a marvellous rest in hospital – that was for the
birds. My brother-in-law is a nurse. He has friends who
are doctors. According to them, I was putting my life and
the child's life at risk.

Joan says she was criticized for her decision by her brothers,
and by friends, especially after what had happened on her third
pregnancy:

I decided to have the baby at home. Everything was fine.

I'd been to the doctor's the day before. He didn't know he was breech . . . I had a midwife booked. We rang her in the morning. She wasn't there. We rang again but we couldn't contact her. I wasn't worried. I knew my labour would be long.

The doctor came at twenty minutes to nine. At ten to nine, he went off saying he had to make a phone-call, even though there was a phone downstairs. He was gone ten to fifteen minutes. I needed a forceps. The flying squad came out from the Iveagh but they got lost. They delivered the baby. The head was caught for three-quarters of an hour. The rest of him was out.

During the night I was given no information. I was told that he had a 50:50 chance. He would have been brain-damaged if he'd lived. He was born at around nine o'clock. He died at three the following morning. I never saw him after [he died]. It shouldn't have happened. He was seven and a half pounds. He was a full term baby.

I just wanted to have my baby at home. It was a dear price to pay. I blame the doctor. It was his mistake. He should have had a forceps with him. That was why he had to go off. If I'd known the baby was breech, I'd have gone straight to hospital. I was relying on the professionals to tell me. If he'd told me in labour, I'd have sat in the car and gone straight to the Iveagh. He didn't say anything. He said everything was fine, that he had to go off and make a phone-call and that he'd be back.

Joan says she would never go near the Iveagh again, not even to visit:

When I was going up in the lift, there were two nurses. They asked me what had happened. They thought first that the baby had just come too soon, but when I told them I'd planned to have him at home, they said I'd no business staying at home. I remember one lady doctor who told me I'd put my own life and that of the baby's at risk by staying at home, that now I had to face the consequences.

Her fourth child was born at home, with the help of another doctor and another midwife. This was her fifth baby and her third home birth: 'I made my decision, and that was it. They didn't make me change my mind.'

The majority of women were constantly being told by everyone how risky it was. 'You're very brave,' neighbours would say. Being told you have great courage can be another way of telling you that you are crazy.

⁓

Psyching Up

How do women withstand the pressure to go to hospital? How do they counter the discouragement, the disapproval, and even the disinformation, heaped on them during pregnancy? Rachel says she got to a point during her pregnancy where she was wavering, 'on the border'. She rang a woman who had had a home birth, who reassured her. Valerie went to meetings on home birth: 'It was helpful, mentally, to hear about other people's experiences.' It made her more determined than ever, she says, to go ahead.

In Ireland, there are about half a dozen birth organizations. Some, such as the Home Birth Centre and the Association for Improvements in the Maternity Services concern themselves with where and how birth takes place. Other groups, such as La Lêche League and the Irish Childbirth Trust, tend to focus on mother and baby after birth. Organizations such as these form an underground web of support, advice and information, and within the group, 42 per cent of women belonged to one or more of them.

Home birth meetings are organized by women for women and men, planning a home birth. Listening to other women talking in someone's kitchen or living-room made the idea of having a baby at home more real, less bizarre. Belonging to a home birth group gave women the feeling that it could be done, that there was nothing to fear, and that it was not irresponsible.

'It's good to know people who approve of what you're doing,' Geraldine points out. For middle-class women, belonging to one of these groups filled that credibility gap – a gap that for less well-off women did not appear to exist to the same extent. If you can remember babies being born at home, you grow up thinking it is normal.

⤳

Words and Pictures

I read Sheila Kitzinger, and lots of other books. At home you have to know more [Carmel].

Women read widely when they are pregnant.[17] Beatrix says she read a lot 'in order to have the arguments ready . . . You have to defend yourself all the way.' Reading is still the only source of information generally accessible to literate women everywhere. The range of books women read was wide, covering everything from the *Chicago Police Force Manual* to Grantley Dick-Read.[18] But this reflects the library stock of the birth organizations. It was through groups like the Home Birth Centre that women managed to get hold of these books. Ina May Gaskin's *Spiritual Midwifery*, Frederick Leboyer's *Birth Without Violence*,[19] any one of a dozen books by Sheila Kitzinger, the same books, the same writers, come up again and again.

Within the group, there are also women who prefer not to know, who avoid everything to do with childbirth, who feel squeamish about 'things like that'. To women with traditional attitudes towards birth, reading books or watching films on the subject bordered on outlandish. Dora says people think too much about these things. She hears women on the radio, she says, talking about childbirth, and they do nothing but complain.

Efa says she would turn off a film on birth if it came up on television. She finds the whole business scary enough as it is.

Only a minority of women watched television programmes or films on birth. Programmes, films and videos on birth, unlike books and magazines, were not widely accessible. Seeing them depended on other people showing them. Films on birth, for example, could only be obtained through the birth organizations.

If you really want to prepare yourself, however, real life is superior to celluloid, as Linda points out: 'I was at the birth of a friend of mine, and that was marvellous, much better than any film.' Hardly anyone else in the group had witnessed a birth.

෴

Learning How to Have a Baby

Attending an antenatal course is one of the accepted ways of preparing for childbirth.[20] Sometimes, it is even set down as a pre-condition by homebirth doctors.[21] Three-quarters of the group did not attend an antenatal course. Most women felt they did not need this kind of instruction. According to Tríona: 'If you've got to go to school to learn how to have a baby, you're in a bad way!' Her view of antenatal classes is that they condition you to have a baby in hospital. Nine women out of ten had given birth before. In addition to ten women with specialist knowledge – former midwives and antenatal teachers – there were other women whose knowledge of pregnancy and birth was extremely detailed. And previous experience of childbirth education could be a deterrent. Rose, a nurse, says the antenatal classes she had attended were awful: 'They were just like knitting classes.' Others were put off in the same way. Sometimes women found courses too inconvenient, for reasons ranging from lack of transport to lack of time. And courses in rural areas were few and far between.

Women who attended courses tended to select those organized by one of the birth organizations. A few went to classes given by independent midwives or physiotherapists, and still others opted for private tuition. Only three women attended hospital antenatal courses. There were no courses for home birth as such.

Breathing, relaxation and birth exercises are what women found most useful. Tips and information on pregnancy, labour and birth were passed around. Women having their second or third baby enjoyed meeting other women. For some, it was a chance to take time out, to focus on their pregnancy, away from the demands of home and work and family. For others, doing a course seemed to be part and parcel of the 'psyching up' process that home birth appears to demand. Going to class could have the same effect as joining one of the birth groups, as Aileen observes: 'The woman who gave the class had had two home births herself. So she normalized my decision to have a baby at home for me.' These courses also gave women access to current ideas about birth, and natural childbirth. And since natural childbirth for some women has come to mean subverting the obstetrical status quo, they reinforced women's desire to stay at home.[22]

Complicated Pregnancies

The vast majority of women reported being in excellent general health, and 91 per cent had no problems of any kind. A small minority – 13 per cent – developed complications during pregnancy.

Bleeding in pregnancy – reported by four per cent – was the most common problem. Bleeding could mean that you were about to lose the baby. Máire lost a lot of blood one night, midway through her pregnancy, but she didn't lose her baby. Netta's was a twin pregnancy, initially. At eight weeks, she had a lot of bleeding. At ten weeks she lost one baby: 'They did a scan. "It's a good job we didn't do a D and C," they said. "There's another baby in there."'

Rita continued to have what she described as 'periods' right through her pregnancy. It was the least of her worries:

> The lump in my breast was getting very big. They told me
> it wasn't malignant, unless it moved in under the arm. I
> had a mini-mastectomy at about three months.

If she had known she was pregnant, she says, she would not
have had the operation at all. She was worried lest the surgery
might have damaged the child. The only medication she was
prescribed during her pregnancy was painkillers for her breast
wound.

Two other women – who went on to have unattended births
– also had surgery early in pregnancy. At four weeks, Jenny had
her appendix removed: 'Doctors said I'd probably lose the
baby.' And at nine weeks, not knowing she had conceived,
Cindy had keyhole surgery to remove the scar tissue from the
site of an old womb operation. The doctors did not know she
was pregnant.

There were the suspected complications as opposed to the
actual hazards. Retaining too much fluid, carrying a baby
suspected of inadequate growth, or having a suspected
placenta praevia – the afterbirth below rather than above the
baby, making normal birth impossible – these worries troubled very few.

Deirdre had a worrying pregnancy, despite not having any
medical complications: at 14 weeks, she came into contact
with German measles. By the end of her pregnancy, her obstetrician had ruled out everything except the possibility that the
baby's hearing might be affected.

Altogether, just nine per cent of women were prescribed
drugs by doctors, ranging from antibiotics for kidney infections to Ventolin for asthma. Some women suffered from
'morning sickness', but hardly anyone was prescribed anti-
nausea pills. Anti-depressants or tranquillizers were prescribed to several women suffering from depression. Two
women, following a number of miscarriages, were given a
course of hormone injections to maintain their pregnancies.

꒱

Quantifying the Risk

In deciding to give birth at home, women feel that they are taking it upon themselves to assume responsibility for the birth. Laura speaks for almost everyone in the group when she says: 'You're taking your life into your own hands.' It is a heavy burden. 'Am I endangering my baby's life?' women asked themselves. Taking responsibility means being accountable for whatever happens. At home this responsibility is all too clear in women's eyes, whereas in hospital, someone else is carrying the can, or so it seems. Penny spells it out: 'We fully accepted that it was our own decision to have a baby at home, and if something had gone wrong, we would have accepted that too.' No one can blame you when you have your baby in hospital.

The additional weight of responsibility is something nearly every woman in the group carried consciously. Chrissie was asked by a hospital doctor if she was prepared to take responsibility for the birth: '"This is a baby, you know", he said. I said, "Yes, it's my baby".' There are women who have no doubts about what they are doing. They are in a minority. Many women in the group had read up on it, and came to the conclusion that there was a very, very small chance that something could go wrong. Jacqueline had a scan at six months, just to be sure the baby was lying in the right position: 'I wouldn't have had the baby at home if everything wasn't normal,' she points out. Neither would anyone else in the group. Women reflect on the risks of having a baby at home: they look at their own health, and they see themselves as healthy. And because they see the baby as part of themselves, because they see labour and birth as a natural process,[23] they feel the outcome is bound to be good. A small proportion of emergencies arise during birth, Sian points out: 'But a trained midwife or flying squad should be able to deal with those.'

Women occasionally focus on specific risks. 'You can haemorrhage at home,' Laura says, 'that's the only thing.' She was having her sixth child. In the days when home births were common and families larger, doctors advised women to have their fifth or subsequent child in hospital. The other big worry women have is, what if the baby doesn't breathe? Women who believe in natural childbirth believe that 'flat' (inert) babies are very rare at home, because of the way the birth is allowed to develop.

So, actually having that baby at home depends on how the pregnancy goes, on not developing complications which would make a normal delivery impossible. In the event of a baby lying across his mother's abdomen diagonally, being able to have a home birth will depend on whether or not the baby moves into a position compatible with vaginal birth. Linda, who was having her second child, had what is called a 'transverse lie' at 37 weeks. The baby turned, but the doctor still was not happy: 'He said if the head wasn't fitting in on my next visit, he would not be recommending a home delivery.' This illustrates just how tight the medical criteria for home delivery can be: in a womb made more elastic by a second or subsequent pregnancy, the baby's head does not necessarily descend into the bony spine of his mother's pelvis before she goes into labour.

Complications were sometimes suspected towards the end of a healthy pregnancy. Several women felt they were being manipulated by their doctors. Sarah's end of pregnancy story is remarkably similar to Carmel's:

> I was anaemic and the doctor used this to try to get me to go to hospital. They said everything was fine. He encouraged it all the way and then at the end, he pulled out. He said I was highly strung. He didn't like the idea of women making decisions.

Two weeks before her baby's birth, Tríona was discovered to have protein in her urine, medically regarded as a sign, if it occurs in conjunction with high blood pressure and swelling of more than the hands and feet, of what used to be called toxaemia. Pre-eclampsia, to give it its modern name, is a syndrome associated with convulsions in the mother. Although her blood pressure was normal and there was no sign of swelling, Tríona was sent by her GP to see her consultant: '"Do you want your baby to be born dead?" he said. I cried. "I'm not having this baby in hospital," I said.'

Having a home birth is not something women do lightly. The difficulty with risk is that, in addition to being a reality, it is also a matter of opinion. Separating the perception from the reality is difficult. Women in perfect health often experienced huge pressure to go to hospital. And women who would have been classified as 'high risk' by obstetricians, were not necessarily discouraged at all.

Only in retrospect can labour be seen to be normal, say obstetricians. The classic argument against home birth all over the world is that since you cannot predict with absolute certainty how things will go, the only safe place in which to have a baby is in hospital. In the late 1960s, obstetricians began to construct risk scores as a means of identifying the fetus at risk. Each obstetrician had his own ideas about risk, so the construction of each score differed.[24]

According to one such score based on the results of the 1970 British Births Survey[25] which measures risk in early pregnancy, one third of the group would have been advised to go to hospital. Using this particular yardstick, it was not difficult to score enough points for hospital.

There was a loading against women over the age of 30, for example; this affected a large proportion of the group – half were thirtysomething. Within the group, the average age was 30.4 years. Women with more than three children were also at a disadvantage. Eighteen per cent of women would have been advised to go to hospital on the grounds that they were having a fifth or subsequent child. Similarly, the nine per cent having their first baby.

The calculation of risk, as the English statistician, Marjorie Tew, has demonstrated,[26] is extremely problematic. A woman who has had several children, for instance, is likely to be older. Much of the risk statistically associated with age is accounted for by family size, and vice versa.

Scores have been criticized on the grounds that they take no account of individual differences. If you are single, for example, or if you are separated or divorced, this is enough to catapult you into the risk category. As many as 20 per cent of the group were technically single, separated or divorced at the time of the birth. The score did not allow for the concept of the unmarried family. If you were working-class, you were defined as being at risk. Within the group, social class loading affected two women in every five.

Being 5 ft 2 in or smaller was another 'contraindication' for home birth, a risk factor. If you were small, then your pelvis might be correspondingly narrow, obstetricians seemed to think, too narrow for the baby to come through. A tenth of the group failed to meet the obstetrical height requirement stipulated by this particular score.

In addition to the social, economic and biological requirements, a woman had to satisfy obstetrical criteria, which related to previous pregnancies and births. Within the group, no one had had a stillbirth, for example. But two women had previously given birth to babies who died within the first seven days of life. Miscarriage was another disqualifier. British statistics showed that the perinatal mortality rates associated with pregnancies following miscarriage were almost double that of pregnancies not following miscarriage. Within the group, one woman in seven had previously had a miscarriage.

Kathleen was having her tenth child at home: 'The doctor said there was some chance my womb might rupture with my tenth, but I said I didn't want to hear any more about it.' One woman had kidney disease, and another suffered from rheumatic heart disease, a legacy from a childhood attack of rheumatic fever. A third suffered from chronic high blood pressure following a car accident some years previously. However, they did not see themselves as being at greater risk.

Other risk factors not addressed at all by obstetrical scores were taken into account by women. If something went wrong, Maura says, she was five minutes' drive from the hospital. For some women, distance from the nearest maternity unit is a major factor in their assessment of the risks involved. The majority of the group lived in cities, half an hour's drive from a maternity unit. You could be in there in the time it takes to prepare an operating theatre, women pointed out.

Thea just did not have that kind of security:

> I knew if there were complications, we would probably have no chance, but I didn't think there would be any. You cannot be frightened.

She was an hour's drive from the nearest maternity hospital. A third of the group lived deep in the heart of the country. Asked if any arrangements had been made with the hospital, just in case, Thea replied: 'No, we understood that if a mother had to go to hospital, she would not be let in.' Few felt as isolated from the health services.

Finding professional help is one of the biggest stumbling blocks women who want a home birth face during pregnancy. Many of those who succeeded in getting a service from the state did so only after a protracted struggle with health officials.

Women who encounter official hostility tend to see less of doctors, going later and less often for antenatal check-ups. Official disapproval only serves to drive home births underground, to a point where a woman will do without antenatal care, or professional help. Sometimes, women see no point in hitting their heads against a stone wall.

Only the birth organizations countered the disinformation, the discouragement and, occasionally, the bullying meted out to women wanting home births. In offering access to current thinking on childbirth to these women, they provided the only counterbalance there was to obstetrics.

𝒳 5 𝒳

Pain and pleasure

It started on Sunday night. It was very mild. It progresses, and progresses and progresses, then it stops. That's the way it always is. It stops at about two centimetres.

The morning before she was born, I went to my doctor. The head wasn't engaged. He said that was no problem. With a fourth baby, the head would engage at the last minute. To be on the safe side, he sent me into the Iveagh Hospital for a scan.

I was getting the odd contraction. There was this tiny screen, and the doctor said 'Can you see the dot?' Of course, I hadn't a hope of seeing it! He said 'I think you'll be having this baby in about two weeks.' There I was in front of him, bent double with another contraction! I asked him, 'What about the placenta?' I wanted to know if it was in the right place. I knew someone who'd had a placenta praevia and I wanted to make sure. He said 'You're very knowledgeable.' He wasn't very nice. On the way out, the same sister I'd had in the Iveagh the first time [on a previous birth] came down the stairs with me. I got another massive contraction. She said, 'All that pulling and poking sometimes has that effect.' I could see John (my husband) waiting for me. He couldn't stop laughing. The sister went red in the face. I could see she thought he was laughing at her. Once we got outside the door, I asked him why he was laughing. He said, 'I must be the only husband in the country who's taking his wife out of the

Iveagh to have a baby.' And we both fell about.

When we got home, I walked the floor. I'd been told by a friend of mine, every time I got a contraction, to squat down a bit, to help push the head into place. I couldn't settle. If I sat down, I got backache. If I stood up, the pains were in front. We walked, talked, watched telly. It got slightly worse. Mrs Kennedy [my midwife] rang at six. I'd contacted her in the morning. She arrived at nine and said 'I'm here for the night.' I was about three centimetres when she checked me. The doctor arrived at twenty past ten, and left again at about half eleven. I was a bit huffed. I'd expected him to be there. 'Don't be silly, Christina,' my sister said, 'You couldn't be in better hands.'

Mrs Kennedy brought me upstairs. John brought up all his papers and wrote out the bills! By one o' clock, I was only four centimetres dilated. She asked me if I would take some pethidine. I was too tired to argue. She said 'It's not for the pain, it will relax your muscles.' I was too tense in the lower regions. I didn't like the pethidine. It was horrible. It didn't do anything for the pain, and it made me woozy in the head. But it must have relaxed my muscles, because half an hour later, she was born.

My sister was outside the door. She heard three screams. When she heard the first one, she said she couldn't stand it. At the second scream, she got up to get her coat. At the third, she was at the top of the stairs getting her gloves! I remember she put her head in the door, she was wearing her coat. The baby was born. And she's in charge of a hospital ward!

All Mrs Kennedy needed was two towels and two buckets. When she broke the waters, she had a towel, and the towel went into the first bucket. The second bucket was for the afterbirth. When she came in, my sister said, 'Where's the mess?' That's all she could remember of her midwifery training! There used to be water everywhere, she said, and blood. 'Cleaning up after them.' Mrs Kennedy just laughed [Christina].

৵

Going into Labour

How do you know when you are in labour? How can you be
sure? In hospital, labour begins, officially, on admission to the
labour unit, not before.[1] Not even if you have been having
regular contractions for eight hours and your waters have
broken. At home, realizing that you are in labour can be a
long, slow process. Efa thought you were supposed to get
stomach pains:

I had an ache in my back. There were jokes all day in the
hair salon. Did you ever go to the bog to cut turf? It's the
way your back feels at the end of the first day, before you
get used to it. That's how my back felt. I thought the backache was a preliminary. I was waiting for labour to start.

At what point do you allow yourself to know that you are in
labour? For most women, going into labour is part realization,
part acceptance that this cramp that keeps coming back, or
that nagging backache that won't go away, *is* labour. Calling a
midwife or a doctor amounts to a decision that you are in
labour. Nobody in the group had a vicious stab of pain like
Meryl Streep did in the film *Heartburn*, right in the middle of a
barbecue: in real life, going into labour is generally low-key.[2]
Polly was cleaning out the cutlery drawer when it happened:

I started about five o' clock in the evening. I was cooking
the dinner. They were a little bit stronger than niggling
pains. I went ahead and dished out the dinner.

Sometimes the burst of energy many women experience is as
good a sign as any that this is it: 'You know the energy you
get?' Hazel asks. 'I got a *spasm* of work, washing curtains and
everything.' Sometimes it was hard to ascertain how women
knew. Eileen just got a feeling she was in labour: 'At ten o'

clock, I had just put the children to bed, and. . . I knew something was wrong although I had no pains.' Her baby was born two hours later.

Margaret was shocked; it started with the waters breaking:

> I was on the phone. I didn't know what had happened – I found myself standing in this puddle. I put down the phone and sat down.

For one woman in ten, this is how labour announced itself. But this could not be regarded as a conclusive sign of labour. Sometimes, the waters broke early.

How did women feel when it finally dawned on them? 'Excited. You can tell what kind of child it's going to be by looking at it. It's like unwrapping a present, only ten times better,' Patricia says. Others felt the same. A third of the group admitted to feeling nervous or apprehensive. Máire felt there was no way out, no escape: 'I was dreading it. I am very nervous. I just knew I had to go through with it. You can't turn back.' For most women, labour was not something to be dreaded. But feelings can be mixed. Dora was pleased, not just because her baby was overdue, but because 'it would soon be over and done with'. Labour is seen as a test.

If her baby is 'overdue', a woman might well be relieved. The 'estimated date of delivery' means there is a magic date on the calendar to watch: 'Those few days after you're due are longer than the nine months put together,' Nora observes. She was 13 days over, and her doctor kept telling her she would have to go to hospital. Sometimes, there is no agreement as to when a particular baby is due.[3] Occasionally, there were disputes between doctors and women about the estimated date of delivery. 'They dispute it with you, as if you were a half-wit,' according to Vicki. 'I suppose that's because they think all women are half-wits!' According to Peter Huntingford, a British obstetrician, duration of pregnancy is not known in up to 30 per cent of women.[4] Asked how soon they knew they were pregnant, some women told me they knew there and then, to the minute, to the hour. Can doctors know better than women?

The longest pregnancy reported within the group was 44 weeks. As many as twenty-one per cent of the group were 'overdue', carrying their babies for 42 weeks or more. This is the limit as far as a lot of doctors are concerned. These women were facing not only the unwelcome prospect of a hospital delivery, but the dreadful vista of an induced birth. Mary was two and a half weeks over. One night, she decided to take the matter into her own hands:

> I got a very mild contraction at half past nine. I had a hot bath, I ran up that mountain out there, and drank a bottle of cider to bring it on! The contractions started coming every hour or so.

Taking a long, brisk walk seemed to work as well as running up the side of a mountain. Other less pleasant methods of bringing it on included drinking castor oil, used by physicians in the nineteenth century to induce labour[5]. Irene resorted to liquid paraffin. Geraldine took caulophyllum, a homeopathic medicine. Her baby was born three hours later. Whatever method women used, it could not have been further removed from the standard hospital induction.

᠀

Husbands, Mothers and Best Friends

Wanting your partner to be there is part of why women choose home birth.[6] As many as 83 per cent of women were accompanied by their partners along the yellow brick road of labour.

Not every woman had a relationship by the time her baby was due. Four women separated from their partners during pregnancy. And two women in difficult marriages – or in marriages that were difficult at the time – refused to allow their husbands to have anything to do with the birth.

Not every woman wanted her husband to be there. For one woman in four, it was not an issue. Women with more traditional attitudes to birth, like Mona, were often ambivalent about wanting their husbands to be there: 'I hadn't decided whether I wanted him there or not. He hadn't said he would or he wouldn't.' Others, like Irene, were downright hostile to the idea. Asked about her husband's role, she replies, 'I wouldn't let him near it.'

Not every man sees childbirth as something that should involve him. 'He thinks it's women's business,' Máire says, speaking of her husband's attitude to birth, and several other women agree. Tríona was hurt by her husband's attitude:

He wouldn't stay with me in labour. I asked a friend to be there. He didn't want to be in the room with me.

Husbands are redundant in childbirth, she maintains. Not every man agreed with his wife's decision to have a home birth. There were a few men who never came round to the idea. Their wives ignored them. Kathleen says her husband was not supportive of the idea at all: 'We're very old-fashioned,' she adds. But it did not seem to be a major problem: she was having her sixth home birth.

Three men allowed work to get in the way. Six hours into Alice's labour, her husband was called away:

The news broke that our ambulance had been hijacked and two of our men held at gunpoint. One was hurt. I just knew I had to do it on my own.

It is a feature of the birth she regretted.

The only other adult present, apart from the professionals, in 70 per cent of births, was the baby's father. Not many women wanted their mothers or their best friends to be there. A sixth of the group, mostly less well-off, urban women, and women living alternative life-styles, asked a female friend to accompany them. And as far as most women were concerned, one friend was about the limit.

Florence's neighbour ended up delivering Florence's baby:

I must have been in labour all day, but I didn't know it. I was very cross with Elaine. She was two and a half at the time. I must have cleaned the bath at least six times. I did all my ironing and put it away. That's unheard of for me! I usually leave it lying around for a day or two after I do a wash. I lit a fire because I was feeling a bit cold, and cleaned it out before I went to bed. 'Make sure you're home before twelve,' I said to Kieran. I put on a wash in the middle of the night, and I went to bed at one-ish. I woke around two in the morning. I was feeling uncomfortable. Marie (my neighbour) woke up at the same time . . . after three o'clock I got up. I decided to have a coffee and a cigarette.

I went upstairs, and by the time I got to the top of the stairs, I was on my hands and knees. I felt something explode inside in me. It was the waters going. I felt something sliding down. It was her. Marie unlooped the cord. She shot out after that, all pink and beautiful. Dr O'Brien came in with his shirt open, his jacket open, his hair unbrushed. 'I don't know why you called me at all!' he said.

Five women wanted their mothers to be with them. Sometimes it was a case of having to. The night Lelia went into labour, there was a storm. Her husband was away, and she was on her own. Her mother felt she had to stay with her daughter until someone – her midwife or her husband – arrived. They could not come soon enough for her, according to Lelia:

She was just dying to get away. She didn't want to be there at all. She couldn't wait for them to come. And I was getting distressed, and she found that distressing, to see me like that.

Maybe the mother-daughter relationship is too close, sometimes, to bear the kind of stress that labour can entail.

Sometimes women were sufficiently close to female members of the family – to a sister or an aunt, to a sister-in-law or a mother-in-law, to want them to be there, but it was not usual. Olive's story is the only one of its kind. She describes how every time she got a pain, her brother got one as well:

> I saw him on the floor. He was doubled up with pain. I thought it was funny at first. Even when I was in the bedroom, and he was in the living-room, it was the same.

They are very close, Olive admits. He is her only brother, and she is nine years his senior. He was very affected by the whole thing, and he is still mad about Cahal to this day, according to Olive. Doctors would call this 'phantom surrogate pain', but it is not mentioned in any of the obstetrics textbooks.

Having your mother or your sister there is one thing, having your children present is a different matter. Nora says the only anxiety she had was whether or not her children should be there. Birth is unpredictable. Bringing in the children means having to play it by ear until very near the end. Only a minority of women – one woman in ten – considered it.

In the event, slightly more children were present than had been anticipated. Noelle's children belong to the majority, to the seven-eighths who were not there. For all they knew about it, they might just as well have looked for the new baby under a cabbage leaf in the garden:

> When the children came in from school, we told them the doctor had brought the baby in a black bag. They really believed it. It was lovely, their innocence!

༄

Not Among Strangers

The vast majority of women had booked both a doctor and a midwife during pregnancy. Only 15 women were under the sole care of a midwife and to be under the sole care of a doctor was almost unknown. When it did happen, it was a case of necessity, as when a midwife broke her wrist two days before a particular baby was due. That first phone call in labour was made, more often than not, to a midwife, but there were doctors who preferred to be called first. And although standby arrangements were made, doctors were in and out, for the most part, keeping an eye on their patients.

Tara says she would have preferred the doctor not to be present, 'if the only people there were people who were really close to me'. She described her relationship with her midwife as good, the doctor she regarded as a stranger. Women wanted a prior relationship with whoever was looking after them. Knowing the name was not enough. Lucinda's midwife had been arranged by her obstetrician. Lucinda did not feel she knew her well enough to want her to be there, and in the last few days, she decided not to call her at all: 'I was afraid she might be talking at me, that she might take over,' she explains. 'I just didn't want the kind of interplay which would be neces- sary.'

The advantages of knowing your midwife have been docu- mented by others.[7] But not every woman knew her midwife, or knew her as well as she would have liked. As many as 20 per cent of the group had no prior contact with their midwives, or not enough, they felt. Doctors sometimes employed midwives directly. And since doctors rather than midwives provided antenatal care, the chances of getting to know your midwife under these circumstances could be slim.

With general practitioners giving women care in pregnancy, women knew their doctors better than they knew their midwives. Ellen explains what she saw as the advantage of knowing her doctor:

> You feel you can ask questions more easily. I know it shouldn't be necessary to know them in order to feel you can ask questions, but that's the way it is.

With two professionals involved, who was seen as being in charge? Women were divided over the question as to who was responsible for their delivery. Philomena says the doctor was only a figurehead. Many women would have disagreed with this view. Some women expressly wished their doctor to be there. 'You feel that little bit safer when he is there too,' Cathy explains. With two professionals involved, what seemed to tip the balance was the nature of the relationship. Women tended to have a strong relationship with one professional or the other, but rarely with both. Sometimes their relationship with their doctor was the stronger of the two. 'He wasn't some stranger,' Cassie says, speaking of her family doctor: 'We'd a great relationship over the years. He could swear at me and I could swear at him!'

That closeness, bordering on intimacy, was evoked more often as a feature of the relationship between women and their midwives. Women sometimes say they were mothered by their midwives. Mona knew her midwife all her life. She was the family midwife:

> I had lots of cousins she'd delivered. She was so lovely, so kind. You wouldn't be one bit afraid. I knew her family. I knew her daughters. It makes a big difference. There was no panic . . . She made it seem so easy. She was able to put your mind at ease.

༄

Having Preferences

Part of why women want a home birth is because they have their own ideas about labour, and these ideas were often discussed in advance with their midwives. They just agreed automatically about almost everything, Statia says, referring to her midwife: 'I didn't want any episiotomy, any drugs or any enema. I wanted him to be put to the breast immediately.' Women assumed, quite often, that procedures that were part and parcel of hospital routine – repeated internal examinations, pubic shaving, enemas and episiotomies – all the procedures that women object to, would not apply at home. Ursula speaks for most of the group when she says she wanted to be able to move around freely during labour:

> To give birth in whatever position I chose. To have the baby with me. To have my husband with me. To do it the way it felt right at the time. Not to have the cord cut too soon. No injection after the birth. I asked the midwife if she used eye-drops, she said no.

Hardly anyone else in the group mentioned eye-drops. They are not used routinely in Irish hospitals. Ursula does not mention pethidine; like most of the group, she would not have dreamed of taking it in labour. Taking long, warm baths is an alternative[8] – one woman in ten thought she might use the bath for relief in labour.

What happens if there is no automatic agreement between a woman and her midwife? There was one sticking-point, Statia explains:

> The injection of ergometrine was something that was her thing. And the fact that I have red pubic hair. She believes people with red hair are more likely to bleed!

Statia decided to let her midwife go ahead with it, rather than challenge her professional judgment. Some women feel there are risks attached to the use of drugs such as ergometrine, which is given routinely in hospital to prevent bleeding after birth, but only a minority of women brought it up.

Not cutting the cord while it is still pulsating is something both Ursula and Statia raise. Almost half of the group bring up preferences such as this, the freedom to move around during the first stage of labour, or to give birth in whatever position seems best. Virginia, who was having her second child, says this time, she felt more able to experiment:

> I wanted to try and give birth standing up. I also thought about being on my hands and knees. I wanted a calm, loving atmosphere. The birth to be allowed to develop as

naturally as possible . . . The light wasn't going to be too bright – we'd no electricity.

Avoiding noise and bright lights is part of a gentle birth. Like others in the group, Aylish wanted a Leboyer birth:

With the lights dimmed, the baby in nice warm water, handled very gently. Not given Vitamin K routinely, like they do in hospital.

Immersing the baby in warm water immediately after the birth is a Leboyer prescript.[9] However, hardly anyone else mentions Vitamin K, which has been linked with leukaemia, an association now disputed.

Having an elaborate set of preferences can be a defence mechanism, as Claire implies:

Gráinne brought up the question of [delivery] position. I hadn't really thought about it. I had great trust in her and didn't feel any need to lay down conditions to protect myself.

The greater the trust, the less the need for advance negotiation.

What happens if there is no agreement at all between a woman and her midwife? Lelia also told her midwife she wanted a Leboyer-style birth:

She just read me the riot act. I just dissolved into floods of tears. She said, 'What's all this nonsense about putting the baby into a bath? He's going to catch cold.' And I wanted to feed the baby immediately. And she went on about mothers who feed their babies constantly during the first 24 hours, and don't let them cry. They don't get enough oxygen, she said . . . As if I was going to cause him brain damage.

It was not a good start to the relationship.

Not many in the group were like Irene, who says she had no preferences: 'I was laxadaisy about it.' She did have one, as it turns out: 'The midwife gave me nothing. I was more alert, not in the twilight zone.' Not being 'too pushed about it' is how a few other women felt, as well. They do not see birth as something you read up on, or go to classes for ('they're only for women with nothing to do'). During pregnancy, they saw no reason to make any changes in their diet. And while the majority of the group wanted their husbands to be present, these women did not. 'Birthing stools, Leboyer methods, didn't interest me,' Jean says, adding, 'I wasn't into that sort of thing.' There are some women who prefer to keep their distance from 'that sort of thing'.

࿓

Managing Labour at Home

At home, where there is no hospital routine, every labour is a once-off. Only two-fifths of the group were being cared for by midwives and doctors who specialized in home birth. Not every midwife had heard that pubic shaving had been largely abandoned by hospital staff as useless. As many as 3 per cent of women had their pubic hair shaved, and 10 per cent were given an enema. With a total of 39 midwives and 59 doctors involved, there was plenty of room for differences in professional practice.

At home, if you could get your midwife or your doctor to agree to it, you could do almost anything. 'She examined me, gave me an injection, and let me have a cigarette,' Betty says, speaking of her midwife. Wanting to smoke is one thing, putting internal examinations off-limits is another. Aileen could not bear anyone to examine her for the last eight hours of her labour: 'I felt there was a no-go area from my chest down. They weren't happy with that but they accepted it.' She was not the only one to put a ban on internal examinations.

At home, the balance of power could occasionally be

delicate. Elizabeth objected to the fact that her midwife donned a white coat, interpreting this as a sign that she was in charge: 'That upset me. She was trying to assert her professionalism. I didn't like that.' Mona does not say what her midwife wore, but she does point out that 'she'd have her stuff with her, but she'd leave it outside'. She goes on to paint a picture of calm, unruffled domesticity: 'She sat, chatting, cutting up gauze. Even my friend was given scissors. My husband was in the kitchen drying his hair. The kids were in and out.' Charlotte describes the same sort of seamless, unobtrusive midwifery care. Her midwife was like a fly on the wall, she says:

> I had no apprehensions. She examined me and listened to the heartbeat. She was family. There was no patient and nurse thing. It was personal.

Anticipating the Worst

> When you've been through it, you know how bad it can be. You know how far it's going to go, but you also know it will come to an end. Nobody tells you, do they, how painful it is? My mother had nine children, and she didn't tell me. If you knew, it wouldn't be so bad [Lorna].

The idea that there is some kind of conspiracy about labour and, in particular, about pain, comes up more than once. The way Denise tells it, it is like an unwritten code of honour among women, a code of silence:

> I remember there was a few of us pregnant at work, and this girl had her baby before me. And when I saw her, she said, 'It's not that bad'. When the next girl came in to see me, I said, 'It's not that bad'. And I was dying!

Your first birth may well influence how you feel about doing it again. Elizabeth says she was afraid: 'The length of the first

labour had frightened me, and I wasn't very confident.'
Women who have had more than one child tend to generalize
about their labours. If a previous labour was difficult, there is
always the anxiety that this one will be the same. On the other
hand, if an earlier birth was a breeze, there is always the hope
that this one will be easy, too.

Having a first child gives raise to other anxieties. Sue felt she
was facing into uncharted waters, that she was faced with the
anxiety of the unknown. Not everyone shared this, however.
Ute was very sure about one thing, that there would be no
pain involved: 'I knew that the more relaxed you are, the less
likely you are to feel pain.' She had had seven or eight miscarriages, the last one just a couple of months before becoming
pregnant with this longed-for baby.

Ashling did not even know you were supposed to have
'pains' when you where having a baby:

> On my first, I had no pains. I was so thick! They [the staff]
> were screaming at me. I couldn't feel any contractions.
> They said, 'You're having a contraction now'. I couldn't
> feel a thing.

Images of birth are all around us – 'shadow-images', Adrienne
Rich calls them.[10] The classic 'Western' treatment of childbirth, with the woman in the wagon screaming in agony, out of
control, in terror of her life, does not inspire confidence. The
fear and the pain of it all, unendurable and intolerable, that is
all most of us can remember.

In the film *Heartburn*, Meryl Streep is shown having a baby.
She might as well be having a heart attack. We see her
writhing in agony on her way to hospital. In hospital, we see
her supine on a trolley, surrounded by male doctors. A doctor
tells her that it's gonna be okay, she's gonna have a section.
Nobody asks questions. There is a second birth scene. Again,
Streep is shown prostrate in labour, a baby donor surrounded
by doctors. The baby is again pulled out from beneath the bed
linen. There is no giving birth. Having a baby, the film is
saying, is having a section.

The experience of pain, Adrienne Rich says, is historical – framed by memory and anticipation.[11] Women who anticipate severe pain in labour suffer more than those who do not.[12] Half of the women in the group anticipated great pain in labour. 'I was in a blind panic,' Catherine admits: 'I had a sense of impending doom.' Anticipation plays a part in the experience of pain just as it does in the experience of pleasure.[13] It is related to anxiety. Vicki says her labour was never *worse* than she expected:

> I was screaming, praying. It was all in my belly. At one stage I felt as if I was going to pass out, that I couldn't handle it.

What if her expectation made it worse?

A third of the group had doubts about their ability to cope with labour. In a film shown on British television on the begin-ning of human life, birth was described as painful, traumatic, dangerous, and – lastly – joyful. Films like this are supposed to be 'factual', 'educational' and 'scientific'. The programme was written, filmed, produced and directed by a doctor, and it was made in conjunction with a number of British maternity hospitals.[14] If women were not led to believe that birth was painful, traumatic and dangerous, would they need obstetrics so much?

Why do women expect to suffer so much? Sometimes, it can be put down to the experience of a previous birth. We are all influenced by our own experience. But the expectation of pain can be created in other ways. By listening to your mother. By reading. Through doing antenatal courses. By joining the birth organizations.

If you are a midwife, lack of confidence can be related to what you have seen – and heard. Aylish explains how she was affected by her experience of working in a large maternity hospital: 'I was worried about the pain after what I'd seen. You could hear these awful sounds coming out from behind the curtains.'

Confidence is a marker for less pain in labour.[15] 'I love

having babies!' Susan says. 'I had faith in my own ability to cope.' Are women who believe they can handle pain more at ease in labour? Just over half the group were very confident that they would be able to cope with labour, including those who anticipated the worst, in some cases. Maude, a psychologist, explains her ability to cope with the demands of labour: 'My mother gave me very positive attitudes to childbirth,' she says.

Feeling able to deal with pain in labour is also related to where you intend to have your baby. Once she realized she was in labour, Hazel says, the fact that she knew she was not going to hospital meant she did not really get worked up. A study by Gunilla Kleiverda[16] found that the majority of women planning a home birth felt that being at home would help them to cope with pain. They were anxious about the possibility of losing their confidence in hospital. Only a small number of women booked for hospital shared this anxiety. Do women choose the place where they feel they can best cope with labour? Or having made their decision, do they feel they can cope best in whatever setting they have chosen?

At home, confidence is essential. For most women, painkillers were not an option: their midwives did not carry any. Being confident or anxious about *coping* with labour is one thing. Feeling confident or anxious about how the labour itself will go is another. Women who believe in natural childbirth have a head start: they often feel safer at home, away from what they see as the dangers of intervention in hospital.

Confidence can also be built on slender foundations. Nuala admits that she was a little worried about the pain, but she was not as worried about the possibility that something might go wrong:

I am so big – I take a size eight shoe! You know the way they always ask you what size shoe you take? They used to tell me I'd have no trouble.

In the days before the pelvis could be measured with instruments, the belief that there was a relationship between the size of your foot, the width of your pelvis and the size of your baby, must have given comfort to many women.

Eileen, a former nurse, was worried about her ability to push the baby out, after what had happened the last time: 'I did feel I was taking on a lot of responsibility, that I had a bad record.' Confidence is a delicate plant. Dympna's was damaged, apparently, at an early age:

> If I had a worry, it was because of what my mother said to me. I used to get a lot of nose-bleeds, and it was the possibility of haemorrhaging.

The possibility of haemorrhaging after birth is one that many women worry about. Pregnant and trying to organize a home birth, Dympna met a doctor who informed her that there was a one in a thousand chance that the baby would not breathe: 'He advised me not to take that chance, to go to hospital. I changed doctors.' These are the kinds of things you do not forget. In labour, Dympna says, she was a bit frightened:

> It was like being in transition for six hours . . . I didn't want anyone to touch me. I didn't know if I would survive. I thought I was going to explode against the ceiling with the pain.[17]

What if anticipation, perception (of danger) and belief in oneself are all related to the experience of pain?

※

The Reality of Labour

There was a first cousin of ours in the house. She'd spent thirteen years in a convent. She thought she could help. When the time came, it was too much for her. She went downstairs and took a swig out of a gin bottle! [Noelle]

Irish obstetricians compare the first stage of labour to a period pain, a cramp.[18] Pain in labour, they say, is 'patently different from the pain associated with surgical operations, or other forms of injury'. How pain in labour is different, or why, they do not say.

Women often talk about labour in terms of what they had been expecting, better or worse. They talk about getting contractions non-stop with no break in between, about contractions that last for a minute or more. Sometimes, not very often, they talk about where they could feel the pain. About a feeling of soreness. Florence says she could feel her whole body being squeezed into this ball:

'O Sacred Heart of Jesus' I said. I could feel the pain coming from my toes up along the insides of my legs, spreading up around my stomach.

Women occasionally talk about getting a backache, and feeling nothing in front. Efa thought the backache was just a curtain-raiser. 'When it gets stronger,' the midwife said to Emily, 'it will be like a period pain.' 'What's a period pain?' Emily said. She had never had one.

No one has ever fully explained why some women suffer in childbirth and others breeze through. Tríona says pain is part of the whole experience: 'You have to tell yourself the stronger the contraction, the more efficient it is.' Is pain always part of the whole experience? A small number of women refuse to define labour as 'pain'. Ute, who is German, emphasizes the fact that pain is a message. Like all messages, as psychiatrist Thomas Szasz has argued,[19] you can take your own meaning from it. Ute says it all depends on what you want to consider pain:

If you are feeling happy or sad, you cry. It's the same thing with labour. The sensations are so powerful you can call it pain. I had a hundred orgasms on Veronika!

She enjoyed her labour:

125

I was lying down, half on my side, drifting. It was beautiful. I was half-dreaming, going into my body, imagining myself to be the baby.

Aileen, who refuses to see labour in psychosexual terms, says she could only describe labour as an overpowering physical experience, very intense, but not orgasmic:

It's the only time in your life when the mind cannot control the body. I actually wasn't able to actively cope with it. My body just went with it. My brain was elsewhere.

Eileen, a former nurse, assumed her second labour would be as painful as her first: 'With the pain, I felt you must try to let the pain happen. To let the pain go through you.' You would think that pain was an outside circuit that the body was automatically plugged into, like an electric kettle, in labour. In anaesthetics textbooks, the patient is the next best thing to an inanimate object, responding invariably to painful stimuli in a way that can invariably be predicted.[20] Western medicine is based on the idea of the body as a machine.[21] Doctors assumed that pain could be measured, like sound, in whatever is the pain equivalent of decibels. Kieran O'Driscoll, who pioneered active management in Dublin, showed – without intending to – the limitations of this approach. For him, the most impressive feature of pain in labour is 'the extraordinary variation in the reaction of different persons to what is in effect the same stimulus'.[22] By splitting off the mind from the body doctors have made pain in labour one-dimensional.

Virginia dislikes the word 'painful':

I would prefer to use the word 'powerful'. I was never overwhelmed by the pain. I could feel him passing through me. It was incredibly intense.[23]

Women who refuse to define labour as pain call it *sensation*. In doing so, they are putting forward an alternative view, one which is incompatible with the decibel theory.

Pat does not believe that pain in labour, 'measurable' pain, is that different from one woman to another, 'but your experience of it is different'. Is there such a thing as *measurable* pain? One woman's twinge is another's agony. Asked how painful their labour was, a few women feel they cannot answer the question. Lucinda tries: 'On a scale of nought to ten, then it would be ten. . . It was like being shot right through, being knocked to bits in all directions.' The majority of women, 58 per cent, found the experience very painful. We live in a culture that is saturated with the fear of childbirth. Have women internalized the message, from television soaps, like *Thirtysomething* to the Old Testament? The idea that pain has a value, and that pain in childbirth is part of the divine plan for women, is rooted in the Jewish and hence the Christian traditions.[24] Some women grew up with the idea that there is merit in suffering. The mother's achievement, Lelia says, is in direct proportion to the pain. She had a screamingly painful labour. According to Adrienne Rich, what we bring to childbirth is nothing less than our entire socialisation as women.[25]

Only nine per cent of women thought labour was par for the course. It was so weird, so peculiar, Efa says:

I had never felt anything like it before. It wasn't pain as such . . . I was awake, conscious. It was very nice, even though it was so difficult . . . My stomach started going in and out. It was extremely strange.

During pregnancy, she wondered how bad labour was going to be. And afterwards, she wondered what all the fuss was about: 'I didn't think it was particularly bad, or particularly easy.' She felt she had been a fool to listen to other people's opinions.

Labour is not a test of endurance for every woman. Some women got off lightly. Twenty per cent of the group had hardly any pain during this first stage. Tara's labour was short, less than an hour. It was not painful at all, she says:

Well, it was like a period, a bad period, but it wasn't

enough to get me into the bath or anything. I thought it was only just beginning.

She put it down to raspberry leaf tea which she had been drinking for the last three months of her pregnancy. Of course, if the baby comes in five minutes, you hardly have time to get out of your clothes.

Chrissie thought nothing of it:

After the first few, you get used to it. They kind of wore off as they went on. At one stage I couldn't feel them, and the doctor said, 'I can see your stomach contracting!' I enjoyed it!

Chrissie did not believe in reading books about childbirth. She had not got the message that it was supposed to hurt. She did not pay much attention to it, she says. Maybe that was the secret of her labour.

Is childbirth less painful at home? women ask. Many think that it is. Kathleen equates the pain of childbirth with being on your own, forced to lie on your back, and injected, repeatedly, against your will:

You're on your own in there. You feel isolated. Lying flat on your back, with all those injections, it's much harder. And no one asks you whether you want them or not. You just get them. I hate injections. It's the needle I hate.

Can we distinguish physical pain from alienation and fear? Rich asks. Jo conjures up a vision of hell, where the pain of labour melts into the pain of being literally tied to the bed:

To be confined is torture. You are then out of control. The worst thing is to lose control. You could get hysterical. To be strapped to the bed would be pure torture.

Separating the pain of labour from the pain of feeling vulnerable, isolated, and powerless is impossible. What Catherine has to say is revealing: 'It was like you were climbing a mountain for your life. You can't stop. I had no fear. I had a great sense of control.'

Mary compares the birth of her first child, born in hospital, with the birth of her second, born at home:

> With my first child, it was completely different. I was given no reason for the backache. They never told me she was posterior. At home it was a hundred times easier. It was pain that I could handle. It was different to the pain in hospital. I was in control. I knew that nothing would be done against my wishes. At home you are not afraid of what they are going to do next.

Both babies were posterior. On both, Mary had a backache labour. Her second child weighed over ten pounds, nearly two pounds heavier that her first. How could her second labour have been so much easier? Other than to say that first labours are generally a bit more difficult than subsequent ones, obstetrics has no explanation to offer. But being told that backache is only to be expected with a posterior baby makes it easier. It gives the backache a meaning. Moreover, being in control means not being afraid of what *they* are going to do next. Maybe we should begin at the beginning:

> I woke up with a good, strong contraction at half past twelve. My mother went off to ring Louise (my midwife) and she came about twenty to two. When she came in, it was like the cavalry had arrived! The contractions were pretty strong by then. She sat on the edge of the bed. After a while, she asked me would I like an internal. She told me I was doing very well, that I was four centimetres. I'd been three centimetres the night before! But the way she said it, she'd make you feel like you were getting somewhere.
>
> The baby was posterior. I knew myself from the way it felt, and I told her. She didn't say something like

129

'Posterior! We'll see whether it's posterior or not when we examine you.' She listened. At home, the baby is more yours. I can't explain it. You're more in control. I could feel the baby, feel her head, see where her bottom was. In hospital, it's more their's.

Louise suggested I get into a position to try and turn the baby (to kneel with my head on the floor). I stayed like this for an hour. Then I had to move. It wasn't comfortable any more. I had a phobia about water in labour, but this time I decided to get into the bath. The pain disappeared completely. It was marvellous. I was totally relaxed. I got backrubs from Louise and from Seán. I was in the bath for an hour or more. I didn't care about being naked in front of other people, and I'm not that kind of person at all!

It was disappointing to have to call the doctor. I was doing very well up until then. I had to get out of the bath before he came. I was hypnotized. He asked Louise if I'd taken something. Louise said I'd had no drugs, that it was self-induced. She told him this always happens on a natural birth. He was a pest! He was walking around swinging that forceps as if it was a candelabra! Louise said I had a very slight cervical lip and she started rubbing me down there. He was quietly panicking. I could hear these whisperings. I was in transition.

I had one leg on Louise's shoulder. I was lying on my side. I was pushing off her. I didn't even realize it until afterwards. Poor Louise! It was a bit hard. I did get a bit dependent, a bit tired. Then Louise suggested I put my hand down. I could actually feel her hair and she was still inside me! I'll never forget it, feeling her hair. Then I could go on. Keep going. The head was born then. That was a relief. It was a bit difficult to get the shoulders out. She was a very big baby. Louise said, 'You're going to deliver this baby yourself.' I said 'I can't.' She said, 'You will.' She got behind me and supported me. I actually lifted her out myself.

The question we need to ask ourselves is, would birth be less painful if women had more control over it?

༶

Coping Strategies

At the beginning of labour, many women simply sat around, doing nothing in particular, watching television, drinking tea. It was all very relaxed. Asked what she did with herself in labour, Noeleen replies: 'I just smoked and chatted. I must have had three hundred cigarettes under the bed!' Rose says there was something nice about staying up in front of the fire. Talking put contractions into the background, she says.

For women whose labours were long, life simply went on as usual, with housework and cooking to do, and children to look after. Many women believe that labour hurts more if you sit and think about it. Scrubbing the kitchen floor, or cleaning out the bathroom, can be a distraction. Women who woke up in early labour often got up, even if it was the middle of the night.

When things got tough, Lelia says, she finally 'took root' in bed. Hardly anyone did so early on. However, the time comes when you can do nothing else and for most women, this time came sooner rather than later. When things got tough, women did things such as patterned breathing, or they walked around, or got massages.[26] At home you could do anything you liked, as long as your professional attendant was in agreement. Having a free mind, Rosemary stresses, is great. She had a whole battery of techniques:

> Breathing, moving around, changing position. Having ice in a towel on my back. It neutralizes the pain, so that it flows along. Not to allow myself to hold back.

Just under three-quarters of the group used some form of patterned breathing, or made up their own. Ute describes the benefits of 'breathing' in labour:[27]

It was not painful at all. Only that one contraction. I was on my own. I said, 'Jesus, there is nobody here.' Nobody could stand in for me. The contraction got the better of me. It was up to me to do it. Then I started breathing again. I used ribcage breathing. I was very spacey inside my body during the birth. I wanted to stay inside, to follow the baby out. I was out of this world before I started to push.

Is there a connection between being 'out of this world' and patterned breathing? Ursula, an antenatal teacher, points out that women tend to hyperventilate in labour: 'So a lot of them experience a spontaneous re-birth. It is to do with the forcing of the outbreath.'

Women were much more inclined to use traditional techniques for coping with labour, such as breathing and relaxation exercises, rather than soaking in a tub of warm water. Many women emphasize how important it is to keep moving in labour. Almost half of the group found themselves standing, walking, sitting, kneeling, or leaning on something for support during a contraction – any or all of these things helped. Some women went for a walk, while others walked the house. Changing position also helped. Deborah, a former nurse, found going on her hands and knees on the floor a great support: 'I don't think I could have coped in hospital, where there was no one to stay with me, and where I'd be flat on my back.'

A few women did pelvic rocking, an idea borrowed from 'primitive' cultures, which has found its way into the literature on birth. As well as relieving back pain, it is said to be helpful in rotating the baby through the spines of the pelvis.[28]

The next most popular technique within the group is massage – often in the form of back-rubs for backache labours – which is reputed to be comforting in labour.[29] Carmel describes the power of touch: 'The midwife's hand was perfect. She was deadening the pain with the pressure of her hand.' A third of the group found this beneficial. But every woman is different. Geraldine says categorically that she cannot bear to be touched during labour: 'I just tend to go into myself. I don't want to be touched. I don't want to be talked to.' A number of women agree.

A few report using another pressure technique – acupressure – pressing the teeth of a comb into the back of the hand, just where the bones of the thumb and the first finger join. Giving yourself a 'pain' somewhere else can be effective.

Ursula believes in the power of water:

The bath was relaxing. It got me so relaxed it nearly stopped my labour. I felt I could cope far better. The contractions were very intense, but I didn't go under. I wasn't lost and at their mercy.

Breathing became a communal activity:

The breathing really helped. They [the midwife and her husband] breathed with me. I felt it into my body, went with the rhythm of it.

Her labour was a joint endeavour:

I got massage. My friend put very hot towels on my back. She really got into the rhythm of it. I had a lot of lower back pain.

Vera used exactly the same combination of techniques, in a different way. First she drove into town with her husband, just to take her mind off her labour. As she was coming home, she says, her body changed gear:

The pain wasn't very bad . . . The bath really helped. My husband rubbed my stomach. A lot of things helped. I managed the breathing fairly well. I was doing it in the car – I didn't need it in the bath. I stayed in the bath a long time.

Taking a long, warm bath in labour has been recommended.

The water is relaxing, and the buoyancy apparently reduces the impact of contractions.[30] A fifth of the group found the bath a godsend. Dympna, however, found it useless, though as she explains 'There wasn't enough water in it, and it wasn't hot enough.' Maybe there is no such thing as a universal panacea in labour, however.

At home women are free to cope with the demands of labour as they please. A small number of women found other uses for water. Some got relief from hot water bottles, particularly in backache labours, while other women looked for cold compresses or ice-packs.

For Leslie, getting into the bath was just a preliminary:

Once I knew it was for real, I got into the bath and stayed in it for an hour. The bath was marvellous, the comfort of it. Then I got out.

As her labour speeded up, she became more and more restless, moving constantly from one place to another:

Once it really started, it was very painful. I wanted to be on my own. I went out. I went round by the trees. I went down into the stables. I kneeled in a little room on my own when I needed to.

This desire to be on one's own, and to be in an enclosed space, was felt by other women. Lorna took refuge in the bathroom:

I just felt like going in there. I don't know why. Our house is very open, and it was the only place that was not open, where it was a bit dark.

There is no one way.

During labour, women relied to a greater or lesser extent on their partners. Staying in touch – holding his hand, for example – mattered to one woman in four. For Penny, looking into his eyes was how she recharged her self: 'It was the eye contact that gave me the extra strength I needed.'

Some men involved themselves physically in the birth as far as they could, breathing with their partners, massaging them, or holding them. But whether they boiled water or did the breathing hardly mattered. What mattered was the fact that they were there. He could keep the humour up, Fay said: 'In hospital, there was no contact between us.' At home, fathers are necessary in a way that would be difficult to imagine in a team setting in hospital. 'He is a very confident man', says Frances, 'and it was probably the only time in my life that I needed to get that confidence from him.'

Aileen says her husband was a buffer between her and the rest of the world:

> I don't know how I would have coped without Brian. You are vulnerable in labour. You want people to keep away. He was physically able to hold me. I was not able to fight for myself . . . He was a bulwark between me and the outside world. He could ward off any interruptions, or intrusions. He made sure that what I wanted was done.

Like a few other women, she feels that even at home, a man's role is to act as a go-between, to be a woman's protector, her champion.[31] Some women need their partners more than others at a time like this.

Finally, mind control techniques going back to the 1960s, to alternative living and alternative health,[32] were used by a small number of women. Visualization is one such technique. Imagining contractions as surging waves, or as mountain peaks, seeing in your mind's eye an image – the opening of a flower, perhaps – this is how women represented visualization. Several women used self-hypnosis. Bridget used meditation: 'I am a spiritual type of person. This goes hand in hand with the type of birth,' she says. Valerie focused on a print of a famous painting by Monet, of poppies. Each woman had her own way of coping with the demands of labour.

Asked what she concentrated on in labour, Joan replies, 'I concentrated on staying alive.' Dora finds the question irritating: 'What would you expect me to concentrate on?' she retorts. 'Flowers? I concentrated on getting on with it.' 'Getting on with it' is a phrase you hear again and again from women with a more traditional attitude towards birth. Dora believes women think too much about these things.

Not all women see birth as a major life event; some see it as something to be got through as quickly as possible. They do not read books or articles on birth; they would run a mile from the birth organizations. These women often seemed better able to cope with labour. Their attitude was nothing if not pragmatic, and their need of techniques minimal.

Not every woman feels she coped well, or coped all the time with her labour. Trudi, at 19, learned that you cannot cry: 'You have to stay calm.' Harriet says she always feels she can manage at first, then she reaches a different stage:

> I growled, went with it. I was making this basic sound. I wasn't suffering the pain. I was aggressing towards it. The more animal I was, the better I felt.

Making noise in labour has become taboo. Few women mentioned it. Harriet saw women in the east giving birth in a different way. Natural childbirth has taught women the importance of self-control. Being in control means controlling the sound that comes out of your mouth. Patricia, who lived in Africa as a child, is unusually frank: 'There was this deep animal grunting coming from me, and nobody was worried.' Others did not feel that they had a right to make a sound. Vicki jokes about it: 'Apart from the screams, the roars and the shouts, it was fine!' Roaring your head off in labour is not socially acceptable. Making noise is tantamount to being out of control.

Some women see labour in terms of the mind being taken over by the body. Máire finds this loss of control almost unbearable:

> It was like going into another world, being taken over by these forces. You have no control over your body, none. That was the most frightening part of it. It always is.

'In labour you are in a different space, almost other-worldly,' Virginia explains. Birth is a mystery. Words are not enough. She describes the value of 'positive thinking' in labour, as a way of coming to terms with what is going to happen, anyway: 'If you think in a positive way about labour being powerful and strong, it helps you to experience and accept the power of it.' Once you start, women say, there is no going back. No one can do it for you. What happens if the pain takes over? Jacintha says she could not move with it: 'I couldn't get my breath back. I was in a sea of pain.'[33] Being locked up in it, being taken over by it, being swept away by it, this is how women describe very difficult labours. Lelia says she tried not to let the tension build up:

> To remember that it was down here, instead of in my face. Not to clench up, to keep some sort of distance from the pain.

It is hard not to be tense and tight, Thea says. She, too, talks about the need to accept, to let go. Sometimes women's ways of coping sound contradictory. You have to control it and, at the same time, you have to let go.

> Pain is something you flinch from, usually. But I wasn't trying to get away from this. I didn't want it to stop. You have to go with it [Linda].

Listening to Katherina, a German woman, it all begins to make sense:

> The last ten or twelve contractions were orgasmic, blissful. I wanted this baby to come out so much. I was saying yes, yes. Oh, yes. I was really positive, really going with it. You melt into it, and it takes you over completely. It was happiness. It was like reaching into heaven. Dick-Read explains it very well. If you are afraid, the muscles close up, and you are going against the contractions, against the opening up of the muscles. That is why

women feel pain, because they are cramped up.

Natural childbirth has taught women the need to exercise mind control in labour, while at the same time releasing physical tension in the body.

✧

Lifting the Pain Away

Labour is a time when women feel particularly vulnerable, especially susceptible to the atmosphere around them. In labour, Anna says, you are completely auto-suggestive: 'You're wide open, raw, vulnerable. All you need is encouragement, total trust in the midwife and the doctor.' Being wide open underscores the need to have complete faith in whoever is looking after you. Once the midwife came in the door, Philomena says, she 'couldn't care less'. Her anxiety lifted.

One of the keys to walking the emotional tightrope of labour, it is said, is a sensitive midwife or doctor.[34] Having a good relationship with them might be a better way of putting it. Half of the group felt they had a good relationship with their midwife. As many as one in eight, however, judged theirs to be poor to mediocre. It was a clear marker for a bad birth.

Knowing your midwife, as Mona sees it, can mean having to handle your labour well: 'When you know someone, you don't want to act like a right baby. You don't want to play on the fact that they're giving you their full attention.' Looked at in another way, when you know someone, there is not the same need for pain to be used as a plea for help, as a signal for attention.

Breathing in unison, physical contact, these are the things women remember. Nuala compares her hospital delivery with her home birth: 'On Ashling, even though I was drugged, it was worse. But Louise, the midwife, was breathing with me. It was a different experience.' Philomena says she did not feel the time passing:

The nurse was smoking. I was going to smoke but I didn't. The nurse and the doctor were slagging and joking me. She expected me to tear down the walls! I blackened her arm!

The warmth, security and ease of a good relationship comes through again and again. Ger describes her midwife as a gift from God: 'She sat beside me, held my hand and lifted my pain away. She was a marvel.' Hannah also describes the power of touch:

She rubbed my back for me. I had a real comfortable feeling when she was here. I can safely say I wasn't in pain. She rubbed the baby out, really. It was terrific.

Lorna says Louise was 'very relaxed and resilient. She takes you as you are, brings you out of yourself. She used to laugh uproariously at my jokes.' Coming to the end of a long and demanding labour, the jokes ran out:

At the beginning of each stage, you're going into uncharted waters. You need someone to encourage you. It's like steering a ship through the eye of a storm. I was hanging on to the bed, but you have to face on into it. Louise encouraged me to push on up the slope. The crowning felt like there was a blowtorch on me. It was like there was this boulder, you had to push through the pain, just when it was at its highest. You felt you had to push and the pushing was making it more painful.

'It was like watching her play the piano,' Lorna's husband added.

❧

Kit Leo

Kit Leo worked on the district in the days when there was a district midwifery service. She spent all her time, Mary says, drinking tea and talking to her husband:

> She came at about three in the morning. She took no notice of me. She didn't examine me at all. She kept talking to Eric. She told him to make tea for her. I had none. I felt nauseous. I began to wonder if she was going to do anything.

Mary was pleased with Kit Leo's style of doing things: 'I think if I was an African woman,' she remarks, 'I'd be happy just to go out into a field alone and have my baby.' (Birth is never quite as simple as this. In these societies, birth is elaborately bound by ritual and tradition, as Sheila Kitzinger has documented in her book, *Ourselves As Mothers*.[35])

Ute, who is from Germany, says Kit Leo took an immediate dislike to her when she visited her during pregnancy: 'I'd read Kitzinger, and she said, "I've delivered two thousand babies. You only read the books".' In labour, things went from bad to worse:

> I started to boil nappies, to get rid of the chemicals. I made my very own personal bed, with black plastic, newspaper, and a cotton sheet. As soon as she saw it, she took it off. She said 'You can't wash out those stains'. But I hate anything plastic . . . She told me to cut sanitary towels. It was like prison therapy!

Under the stress of labour, latent conflict can easily erupt into open hostility. Ute's birth story becomes an account of a pitched battle between herself and Kit Leo. They were a world apart in terms of age and ideas.

Such differences can exist, and often did, between women and their midwives, without leading to battles in labour. Angela, from Dublin, shares many of Ute's ideas on birth, and on life in general; her experience of Kit Leo, however, was very different:

> We made tea, had a couple of jokes. I breathed through the contractions. She mucked in. The focus was on me. . . She has a real feel for the way a baby is born. It was a piece of cake. It was only for the last two contractions that I got unhooked. In hospital, I was unhooked right through.

Choosing the right midwife can turn out to be the most crucial labour strategy of all.

$\backsim$

Mind-altering and Other Drugs

According to a French psychologist, Claude Revault d'Allonnes, we live in an anti-pain society.[36] Pain is considered to be bad: it is to be combated, and, if possible, removed.[37] The medical response to pain is to control it. Obstetrical textbooks assume that most women require pain relief during labour. In the Netherlands, only a minority of women get drugs for pain relief in labour.[38] According to a comparative study, American women expect birth to be more painful than do Dutch women, and they need more pain-killers in labour.[39]

The vast majority of women in the group – 83 per cent – went through labour without either pethidine or gas. Hazel does not like drugs. She says she would have to be very much in need to take them:

> You're much more alert without them. Pethidine makes you very dopey. I would hate to be like that, not to know what was going on. All drugs have side-effects. Doctors tell you they don't, but they do.

A third of these women knew that, regardless of how it was on the night, they were simply going to have to do without. Drugs were not an option, Agnes explains, because the midwife does not carry any: 'It was just as well, because at one stage in labour I'd have taken anything she gave me.' If you book an independent midwife, you are opting for natural childbirth. Home birth midwives do not usually carry painkillers.[40]

Had pethidine been an option for all, it is doubtful if it would have been in greater use. As many as 88 per cent of the group are opposed to the use of drugs in labour for pain relief. This is part of a world-wide trend. In Auckland, New Zealand, home birth means *natural* birth,[41] just as it does in Salt Lake City, Utah.[42] But there is more to women's opposition to painkillers than a belief in natural childbirth. Some women had had a bad experience of pethidine on a previous birth. Women also have other reasons. Rose, a nurse, was hoping not to have pethidine:

> I wanted to experience labour totally. Pethidine makes it unreal. It takes away from the satisfaction. I felt I could cope. It might affect the child. It is difficult to know when to give it.

For a feminist like Helena, her opposition to drugs is rooted in her need to retain some control. Her labour was very intense, but taking drugs did not arise:

> If I was drugged, I'd be more likely to be taken over, to be done to. I wanted to participate. If I was dopey, I wouldn't have been in control. If you have drugs, you are not able to push.

For many women, there is the knowledge that drugs harm the baby. For women who believe in natural childbirth, the crossover effect is at the core of their objection to pethidine. Lelia says she just needed someone to hold her hand:

That's all. I didn't want to take anything which would affect the baby. If there was a method that had absolutely no side-effects, I would use it, but at the moment, there isn't.

Not every woman has a view on drugs for pain relief in labour. Dora says she left it up to the doctor to decide: 'He knew what he was doing.' Vera's midwife had difficulty in getting pethidine, but Vera was not too worried: 'I said I'd prefer to do without. In for a penny, in for a pound! I thought I'd be able to handle it.' A few women have a fear of needles. Kathleen did not want pethidine because of this, but she was not against painkillers in principle: 'Nurse Cotter had this cloth, and she'd put this blue stuff on to it. Do you know it?' she asks.

Of the group, 10 per cent of women took pethidine in labour. 'The rest that I had with the pethidine for twenty minutes was pure heaven,' Catherine maintains. Women with a more traditional attitude towards birth have more liberal views on pethidine. Jean says it took the edge off the contractions: 'I wanted to have it pretty natural.' Everyone has their own idea of a 'natural' birth. Beatrix, a believer in natural childbirth, was sorry she took it: 'I was nearly there but I didn't know it. If the doctor had told me it would not be long, I would not have taken it.'

Pethidine works for some, but not for all. You need to believe in it, by all accounts. Denise was petrified of the pain: she got two injections. 'They didn't work,' she says. Pethidine doesn't work for me.' Believing in the power of pethidine could be complicated. It was difficult to separate Mona's belief in pethidine from her faith in her midwife: 'She made me feel very easy. She wouldn't leave you in pains. You would get something. Pethidine does relax you a little. I had great faith in her.' Her midwife had worked on the district. That anyone took pethidine reflects the fact that the study is nationwide, that there were different styles of midwifery practice. Midwives who belong to an older generation, who worked on the district in the days when there was a district service, are not necessarily anti-drugs as are the younger, independent midwives.

And not every doctor realized that it was possible to survive labour without pethidine or gas. Olive says her back felt as if it was to come off:

> I wanted to be by myself. I could bear the pain better on my own. He wanted me to have an injection. I didn't want it. He said he would give me half a dose . . . I fought pretty hard against it. I wasn't too happy about the injection, being honest about it. He said it would be better for me. He kept trying to give me gas. I wouldn't take it . . . I didn't want it. It makes you sleepy and dopey. I wanted to enjoy it.

At home, if you felt you needed a painkiller, the only other option was gas. Ellen says she did not know how she was going to manage without the gas. She had used it on all her hospital births: 'I asked the doctor about the gas, but it had been so long since he'd used it, he couldn't even find it.' Access to gas – like pethidine – depended on who was looking after you. Only four per cent of the group used it. Some women who would think twice about using pethidine think nothing of using gas.[43] Cassie says she never took anything in case it would damage the baby: 'I knew I was going to use gas.' She had used gas continuously for three hours on a previous home birth. Like others, she found it took the edge off the contractions.

A small number of women used homeopathics, but arnica was the only one used as a painkiller. Other women, believing that it makes labour easier, took large doses of calcium. Freda says the pain was very strong. She got homeopathics, tissue salts and Bach flower remedies from her midwife, but 'there is no instant relief'.

Claudine, having her fifth child at the age of 40, sees pain in labour as inevitable. She presents her home births as a progression in pain control:

> With Canice, I said please have something if I need it. With Rory, I said only give it to me if I ask for it. With Ciara, I said I did not want anything. I was never at a point

where I would take something . . . It was self-hypnotism . . . If I had three more, I suppose I would be able to have a pain-free birth.

Claudine believes women must not be dependent on others to do it for them, that they must do it for themselves.

ॐ

An Uncomplicated Birth

I went into labour at nine o' clock at night. The contractions were ten minutes apart. I phoned Margaret Sheerin, the midwife, immediately. (She was going to spend the weekend I was due with her sister, so she could be on hand.) She got here at half past ten, and examined me. I was one centimetre dilated.

We were having a dinner party and Bob's friend refused to go home. Margaret said things would probably not happen during the night. She slept in the spare room. I was awake all night with contractions, and with excitement. I was in very good form. I handled the contractions very well. I fell asleep for four or five minutes, then woke up with a desperate contraction. I used hypnotherapy to help me with my contractions and it was great. I made sure I didn't fall asleep again.

In the morning, we had breakfast. She examined me then, I was only two or three centimetres. There was no point in her staying. She would phone at lunch-time, and she would stay with her sister, or come, whichever. The morning went. The contractions were four or five minutes apart.

She phoned at one o'clock. I asked her if she was coming back. She said she would play tennis, and have her tea. 'You can phone me when the contractions are two or three minutes apart. If nothing happens, I'll come back at six, anyway.' She told me to do what I normally do on a

Sunday. I usually go for a walk or read the papers. With these contractions . . . I felt it was obvious that she had never had children. There is a great deal of emotional dependence on the midwife.

I got depressed at about three o'clock. Nothing was happening. I was beginning to feel exhausted. I said maybe it was a mistake to have a home birth. I was very tired and felt I couldn't go through another night. I thought about ringing the Iveagh, but decided I would try and hurry it up instead. I had a bath, and did exercises. The contractions speeded up. They were coming every two or three minutes. I cheered up.

At about five o'clock, Bob was just going to phone when she arrived. They were coming every minute. She came upstairs and examined me. I was seven centimetres dilated. She asked me if I wanted my waters broken. She tried first with her hand. It didn't work, so she asked me if I would allow her to use an obstetric instrument. The waters broke immediately. I got a very strong contraction. I was very excited, very happy. It seemed to me, subjectively, that the baby was born very quickly. I felt that it was only twenty minutes. Objectively, it was about an hour.

When she felt I was ready to deliver, I was to adopt the delivery position of kneeling with my hands on the chair. She said, 'Tell me when you feel the urge to push', which was very different from my delivery in Green Street, where they told me to push before I got the urge. It was dreadful and the baby wasn't ready. I was in bed when I got the urge to push. She put her overall on, and helped me out of bed. Then there was a knock at the door, and the GP arrived and ran upstairs. He was very excited, as his own wife was due in two weeks. He said he had never seen someone in delivery so relaxed. I was chatting and dabbing my head with a cold cloth. The delivery took about fifteen minutes, but subjectively, I felt it was shorter. I was keen not to tear so I didn't want to push too hard. I panted during each contraction and the baby came out very slowly. I did push the third time and the baby's head was delivered, and then all the rest of the baby came in two minutes. She asked Bob did he want to deliver the baby but he said no, so she caught the baby.

Then she pretended she couldn't see what sex the baby was, so she asked Bob to see. She asked him if he wanted to cut the cord, but he said no. She was quite disappointed. She was very much for paternal involvement. So she cut the cord and then the baby started bawling her head off. I was quite surprised because I was so relaxed. I suggested then that the baby might like a bath of warm water. So Bob and the doctor rushed downstairs and filled the ordinary bath. I said no, they had to bring the baby bath up to me. I didn't want the baby taken away at that stage. As soon as the baby was put into the baby bath, she stopped crying, and opened out and relaxed.

Then they opened a bottle of champagne. After ten or fifteen minutes, the midwife pushed on my tummy a little to help deliver the placenta, and it came away. Again she asked Bob if he wanted to see it and he declined. But I did. It was like a lump of liver.

They wanted to be sure she was feeding normally. I was in bed by this stage. The doctor and the nurse checked quickly that everything was normal, and wrapped her. She was put to the breast. Then, when they felt she was sucking, they just went downstairs and left Bob and me alone. The baby was delivered at eight o' clock. She stayed in bed with me. She was sucking all night.

ॐ

Complicated Births

I was prepared to go into hospital if there were any complications, if the cord prolapsed, or there was bleeding or the baby's heart went down [Katherina].

The vast majority of the group – 80 per cent – had no medical complications whatsoever during the first stage of labour. Penny describes how 'The contractions would come, stay for a while and then go.' Looked at medically, this was the most frequent complication of all, reported by nine per cent of the women. Statia says if you sit around, if you switch off, you can get it to stop: 'I wasn't really concentrating on the labour. We sat by the fire chatting. The labour slowed up. It got weaker and weaker.' It was bad management, she says, on her part: 'I hadn't been having enough rest towards the end [of pregnancy] . . . I didn't want to be in labour.' Eileen also blames herself for the fact that her labour slowed up:

I let the doctor and the midwife restrict me. What I wanted to do was to sit on the toilet, and to walk around the garden, and to listen to the drums. They got very anxious if I left the room, and I felt I had to sit with them. I didn't take charge . . . I felt they were just waiting for me to get on with it, and that I was holding them up . . . I could have taken more control. The contractions would have been stronger.

She was slow to dilate as well, and there was meconium in the waters. It can happen when labour slows down. Five women in the group reported that there were signs of meconium. Aileen says the midwife rushed the delivery in the end: 'She was worried about the baby, because of the meconium in the waters.'

Bleeding in labour may – or may not – mean that the after-birth is detaching itself from the wall of the womb. Five women say that they had some bleeding during this stage of labour. 'The bleeding was like a period,' Betty says.

Laura, having her eighth child, developed a swelling on her cervix which was troublesome:

I had an oedema. It was the pressure from the baby's head. It was just at the opening of the cervix. It was very, very sore.

There was a possibility, she says, that she might have haemorrhaged.

Two women say their waters broke early. The waters act as a
barrier to infection. If they go 24 hours or more before the
beginning of labour, there is a risk of infection. Unlike the
actual hazard of an infection, the fact that the waters go early is
not a problem in itself. These first-stage complications are
markers for more serious things that could go wrong later on.
And what is regarded as a complication in hospital may not be
regarded as a complication at home.[44] At home, where there is
no 12-hour limit on labour in force, if contractions slow down
or even stop altogether, it is not necessarily a signal for intervention.

What is regarded as a complication by women may not be
regarded as a complication at all by doctors. Having an 'anterior lip', for instance, is not classified, medically, as a complication. As far as women are concerned, it is a different story. If a
woman pushes before her cervix is fully dilated, it may become
swollen, and this anterior lip can slow up the birth. Rose, a
nurse, explains that she found her labour difficult, because she
had a thick lip on her cervix: 'I was not fully dilated, and I had
to work hard to deliver the baby.'

᠄

Sprints and Marathons

How well you cope with the demands of labour can depend on
how long it lasts. A quarter of the group got off lightly, taking
less than three hours, by their own estimation, to get to the
pushing stage. Women occasionally remark that they must
have been in labour all day without knowing it. Or else that
they must have gone through it in their sleep. Just as doctors
believe labour must be painful, so women believe it has to be
long.

Patricia believes that a short labour is just as demanding as a
long one:

With a fast labour, it is a sprint rather than a marathon, but I think you put the same energy into it, in terms of units, as someone else who has a much longer labour.

She had a two-hour labour. But a short labour does not have to be screamingly painful, any more than a long one has to be exhausting. When she awoke, Thea says, she did not know whether she felt like making love, or whether she was in labour: 'I decided to get out of bed, and then I would soon know! The cows had to be milked and the animals fed. I wanted to be on my own.' She got contractions at seven, the boys were sent out for the midwife at eight, and her daughter was born at nine.

Rita, having her sixth child, had the shortest labour of all:

I just got a pain in my hip, went upstairs, and went down on my hands and knees, and the next thing I had to get my tights and pants off. One pain, one push and there she was. I didn't even know the head was born.

As it is difficult to know when labour begins, how long it lasts is a matter of opinion. That first ache – if it does not go away – is the beginning of labour. Women see labour as a state of being, which once entered into, only comes to an end with the arrival of the baby. The fact that during labour, they might bake bread, or go for a walk, or have a swim, makes no difference. Estimating labour from first twinge to first push can make for long labours. Joan says hers started at about six o' clock in the morning, with niggly pains:

I thought the pains weren't severe enough. It started in the back, then moved to the front. I had a show during the day. I remember standing at the twintub doing the washing at six in the evening. It started to build up then. I was standing up against the radiator for about an hour. He was born at around nine.

Asked how long her labour was, she replies it was 15 hours.

Obstetricians would have said she had a three-hour labour. Another woman says she had a 17-hour labour, ignoring the fact that she went out of labour altogether for 12 hours.

The women tended to have short labours. Calculated by doctors, the average labour within the group would only have been three and three-quarter hours. By their own estimate, almost half of the group were in labour for less than six hours. This was just as well for all concerned. However long labour lasted, women preferred the midwife to stay. In the event of a 24-hour labour, there was no one to take over. Less than a third of the group, according to their own calculation, had to cope with labour for longer periods – between 6 to 12 hours. So much for the books that said your first labour would last for 12 hours, and that, on a second baby, you could expect to be in labour for 8 hours at least.

Cassie had a 19-hour labour, with 'iggly' pains for the first 6 hours, before it became harder:

> They came so quick I couldn't manage the gas. They'd have sectioned me if I was in hospital. It was very, very strong. Very, very long. I remember looking at the wall-paper, and wanting to tear it off. Then I thought, 'I can't do that. We've just papered it.'

Labour in excess of 12 hours is said to be 'prolonged', and is classified by obstetricians as a complication. Their solution is to accelerate it.[45] Anna finds this unacceptable. A long and arduous natural labour, she feels, is better than a short one which has been 'stimulated' with oxytocin:

> In hospital, I would have been put on a drip. That would have taken away my control, I would have had to have painkillers, and then I might have needed a forceps.

None of the women had their labour accelerated by drugs. A minority, 19 per cent, had their waters broken, a procedure often used routinely in hospital to speed things up. Christina explains that her midwife thought they were ready to go, anyway:

I was only five centimetres dilated. If she hadn't broken them, I would probably have been here till nine o' clock in the morning.

Hilary's experience was less positive. She was just beginning to deal with the contractions when the obstetrician broke the waters: 'It got much heavier. He asked me if I wanted something, but he told me it's gonna make you drowsy. I didn't take anything.'

Going over 24 hours was unheard of, but for 20 per cent, who said they were in labour for 12 hours or more, labour was long. Six hours is the cut-off point, according to obstetricians. They say the morale of the 'average' woman begins to deteriorate visibly after 6 hours: 'After 12 hours the deterioration accelerates rapidly – in geometric rather than arithmetic progression almost – until, eventually, a stage is reached at which an adult woman is reduced to pleading for deliverance, unless she is rendered semi-conscious with drugs or lulled into a false sense of security with epidural anaesthesia.'[46] This theory – which has influenced a whole generation of obstetricians – is not borne out by the present study. Nobody's morale collapsed, geometrically or any other way, in a long labour.

Nora's story shows the need for nuance when we talk about labour:

There was a regatta on, and we went for a walk. That night, at ten o' clock, I was seven centimetres. It had taken 24 hours for me to get from three to seven and I'd no pains, no sensation whatsoever. I'd been three centimetres since I was seven months. My mood changed – I went more into myself. I was feeling very uncertain. At six o' clock in the morning I woke up. I was terribly disappointed that I was not in labour.

We did some weeding. It was a fabulous July day. We went to the cathedral and said a prayer. My mood was changing. I got very introspective. I wanted to go home, to be on my own, to be by myself. At five minutes to one, she examined me and I was ten centimetres. And I hadn't had any sensation at all, not even a twinge.

Pain and labour are not always the same thing.

ॐ

In 'Transition'

This was like an expulsion from the body . . . the speed, the strength, the power in my body. It was a tremendous experience. I felt as though I could take off into outer space. I was propelled into space [Lucinda].

'Transition' is the name given to what is seen as a distinct and particularly difficult phase at the end of the first stage of labour, before the beginning of the second stage. Harriet says she does not have easy births: 'They don't just pop out. I get het up in transition.' For a third of the group, this is when their waters broke. But the breaking of the waters is not what we usually associate with transition. In the birth literature, transition has been characterized by strong, frequent contractions, trembling, nausea and vomiting.[47]

Tara gives us a picture of transition rarely found in books. She describes it very positively, in terms of heightened awareness, something some women experience in labour: 'I felt physically that my eyes were very wide open. Transition was amazing. I felt really alive and aware. Very good about it, and strong.'

Within the group, transition was a minority experience. Brenda had to wait for five hours while the baby came down through her pelvis, but she did not see herself as having been in transition:

Once I was ten centimetres dilated, there was a long delay before the baby was ready to emerge. Dr Brennan said this was because he was still high up in my pelvis. I just waited and waited. The baby just descended in the end. After five hours, I pushed. Just two pushes and he was out.

Most women did not experience it at all as a distinct stage in labour. The idea of *transition* is unknown to women who have not come into contact with it in books and magazines. This does not mean that they may not suffer extreme pain, or lose control. But these women did not classify these as symptoms, because they had no concept of transition as a distinct stage in labour. The question we need to ask ourselves is, do they suffer less?

Kathleen, having her tenth child, had never heard of transition. As far as she was concerned, it was time to call the midwife:

I don't like fussing. I don't believe in panicking. She'd only be here about half an hour before the end. There was no point in the two of us just sitting there, looking at each other. You're better off without [them].

Like a few other women – mostly less well-off, urban women – she had complete confidence in her own ability to bear a child.

༄

Giving Birth

I was still in my clothes. I flung off everything I had, and got into a nightdress. My friend had gone off to collect another friend of mine, who was a midwife. Margy was still in the kitchen. I was standing up beside the bed, holding on to this head. I called her to catch the baby. 'Mind you don't let it fall,' I said. 'It's going to be very slippery.' Between us we got it on to the bed. There were lots of newspapers around, and I told Margy to put them on the floor, before the carpet got destroyed! I told her where to find the [maternity] pack. She couldn't find scissors. I clamped the cord and cut it. The afterbirth came quickly. I had a flannelette sheet airing in the hot press. I told her to get it and put it round the baby. It was only then I asked myself what had I?

Susan, a nurse, gave birth to a baby daughter.

Virginia, who is English, tries to explain exactly what is involved and how it feels:

It's not pain. It's a different feeling, an overwhelming pushing sensation. It's a very physical experience. Your whole self is involved [she makes a rippling motion with her hand, from the top of her head to the soles of her feet] trying to push the baby out.

There is not always an impulse to push. A number of women gave birth without having any physical urge to do so. Some feel they had to work harder as a result, others describe how the baby just slipped out all by herself. Maeve says she began to push just as the baby's head was coming out:

I was on all fours. Hanora, the midwife, was behind me, my husband was in front of me, and my sister was beside me. I just gave one almighty push, and Sorcha shot out. Hanora just about caught her.

Women occasionally present successive labours as a learning curve. Valuable lessons can be learnt during the second stage. Fionnuala says it was not until she had Emer that she made the connection between pushing and tearing: 'I learned not to push so hard.' Ursula says she just needed to give herself time:

During the delivery, I grazed the front of my vagina, then I tore towards the back. Both shoulders came together – it was too quick. He was crying inside. I could hear him – it was too expulsive. The graze was nasty. I should have held back.

Patricia feels that despite having had two previous hospital deliveries, her body had not been given the opportunity to learn how to do it. Getting him out was a bit difficult, she says, more than a bit difficult:

> When the head was crowning, I thought 'I just cannot do this.' The body has a memory. After two episiotomies, the body wasn't in tune. Being on the horizontal meant that it hadn't experienced the weight of gravity. It was that feeling of stretching – someone described it as a burning grapefruit. His head was like a rugby ball, and he was very big.

The pleasure of an easy birth, feeling your body wide open, letting this baby slide through you, can be infinite. Some women cannot bear the idea of giving birth. The end – as these women see it – is often the worst. Sarah, another nurse, says it is the most frightening part of labour: 'At the end I feel as if I am being torn apart. I always feel that. I think it's normal.' It is the opening up of the body involved in the crowning of the baby's head that is the worst feature of it for some women. Katherina demonstrates why she found it painful: 'If you do this [she extends her thumb outwards as far back as she can from her hand] you feel a tingling sensation here [in the valley between her thumb and her index finger.] That is the way it felt.'

Why do women fear giving birth? Claudine, from Switzerland, believes that it is difficult for women in the West: 'It is an area of the body we are not comfortable with.' Not every woman is prepared to talk about the second stage of labour in any detail. Is it more difficult for women in Ireland, brought up in a culture where even the blood of menstruation could hardly be acknowledged? Or is it difficult for women in the West, because contemporary Western culture has made its own special contribution to the alienation of women from the birth process?[48]

Sometimes there is a physical reason for the difficulty: 'The baby should have folded in his shoulders,' Ger explains, 'but he didn't.' More often, it is the uncomplicated births, the ones where there was no physical reason for the difficulty, that were the worst. Denise is one of the few who felt she could not do it, not just initially, but for what seemed like forever:

> She told me to push but I couldn't. I had no urge to push. I couldn't bear lying down so I got up. I remember going over to the window and standing there. The flows of pain were stopping me. At one stage, she said to me, 'Do you want to have a dead baby?' I didn't like that. My husband said, 'I think we'd better phone the Iveagh.' And she said, 'Yes, maybe you should.' When I saw the ambulance outside the door, I thought, 'That's it. I'll have to do something. It's now or never.' She came out so easily. I'd found it very painful on my left side. Standing up, it was brilliant.

It was a three-hour labour, without complications, that Denise saw as a nightmare. 'The midwife told my husband, "She is fighting those injections [pethidine]." My husband was concerned. He was even more nervous than I was.' Denise, hindered by her own lack of confidence, a midwife who did not give her support, a husband who did not think she could do it, was saved, finally, by the discovery that standing up was brilliant.

Nervous husbands were no use. What women felt they needed at this time was support and encouragement. He needs to have faith, too, according to Elizabeth, to feel that you can do it:

> He was crucial, completely tuned to what I wanted. He took all the abuse! He was very supportive. When I was pushing, I was leaning against him – he was sitting behind me. You can't do it on your own.

Not many men involved themselves in the birth to the extent of physically supporting their partners in this way. A few men simply did whatever the midwife asked them to do: several 'caught' the baby at her invitation. Most were content to be this bulwark of faith, hope and confidence that many women so needed at this time.

What happens if the midwife does not make it in time?
Niamh was asleep with her two-year-old daughter on the floor
of the living-room, in front of a big, open fire. She had been up
with her all night:

> I woke up at six o'clock. I had a sandwich. Went to the loo.
> Had a show. My neighbour, who's a nurse, came in. We
> had to go out to phone Kit Leo, the midwife. She asked us
> if she could have a cup of tea, and said she'd be round in a
> few minutes. When I got back, I got into bed. I felt the
> urge to push. By the time the midwife arrived, the head
> was born. The baby just fell out. She was born at ten to
> seven.

Niamh was not the only one who had to manage on her own,
when the time came, despite having booked a midwife. Eleven
per cent of babies arrived before the midwife or the doctor.
Many of their mothers had short labours. If you have a 50-
minute labour, and you have booked to go to a hospital 50
miles away, your chances of having professional help may be
equally slender. Also, there were a few women who wanted to
manage on their own for as long as possible. Jean, like
Kathleen, says she would hate the midwife to be sitting
around, so she left it until as late as possible to call her. With
arrangements like this, it was inevitable, sooner or later, that
the baby would come first.

If the baby comes first, his father may have little choice but
to deliver him. Most men who acted as midwives did so by
choice. Others got caught out. Terry's husband could not find
a public phone in the neighbourhood that worked. He ended
up getting a taxi-driver to phone the midwife, but by the time
he got back, it was too late: 'He guided the baby out so that it
wouldn't flop on to the floor, off the bed,' Terry says, calmly.

At home, taking a more active role could be a case of necessity, as Noeleen points out:

> He held my legs, that was about all! I always remember
> him standing there looking straight ahead at the wall. 'You

can do it,' that's all he said! He hardly knew which end the baby came out of! He wouldn't have been there at all, but he'd no choice. He's not that kind of man.

Ashling had to manage with only her aunt, who had not even wanted to be there, for support. To make matters worse, her waters had not broken.

It was ten to eleven, the midwife still hadn't come. My aunt kept on looking out of the window. She said, 'Don't have the child yet.' I was roaring. The water bag came down. I didn't know what it was. I thought it might be the head, but it was all soft. My aunt said, 'That's only the water bag.' Then it burst, and I got into bed. She was over at the window when the head came down. I said, 'You'll have to come over,' and the rest of him came. 'Make sure the cord isn't around his neck,' I told her. She caught him.
Then Kit Leo came. She delivered the afterbirth. She rang the doctor and said DOA. I thought it sounded like 'Dead On Arrival!' I had one stitch. The doctor had a brandy afterwards. My aunt had to have a brandy as well. She was all shaking and rattling. 'What about me?' I said.

It was rare for the waters to be intact at birth: only six women reported it.

ॐ

Doing It As You Please

Outside the confines of hospital delivery suites, left to their own devices, how do women deliver their babies? Two-thirds of the group gave birth lying down, or semi-propped up, in bed. Patricia reacted strongly to the colour of the sheet: 'There was a white sheet on the bed. I didn't want to get on to it. The white sheet looked too painful. White is a very hard colour.' She had had a bad hospital birth. A few women opted for what is known as the 'left lateral' – lying on your left side. This has become the position now favoured by obstetricians since the demise of what has been called the indelicate lithotomy – or stranded beetle – position.

Other women gave birth sitting upright (on the edge of an armchair), kneeling, on their hands and knees, or standing up. Several women changed position during the birth, delivering the baby's head in one position and the rest of his body in another. A few women felt constrained by the fact that their midwife was elderly; they were reluctant to take up a position that would require her to bend down or to go on her knees. Agnes is one of the few who squatted: 'I was in a supported squat, with my husband holding me from behind. The bond with the baby is better.'

༈

The Baby Makes a First Appearance

Nature was kind. Almost every baby was lying in the right position for birth, and in 88 per cent of cases, the baby's head had already 'engaged' or descended into his mother's pelvis.

A lot depends on how the baby makes her first appearance. The vast majority of babies (91 per cent) appeared face down, with the tops of their heads showing. This is the most usual – and the most favourable – position for birth. Any other form of appearance is considered, medically, to be a 'malpresentation': the measurements of the baby's head are wider coming through the birth canal, making the birth potentially more difficult. Also, there may be no 'moulding' of the baby's skull – when the bones slide under each other to make her passage through the birth canal easier. Malpresentation is associated with larger families; the baby has more room to move inside a womb already stretched by several pregnancies, and this increases the chances of her getting into an awkward position.

Four babies were born face up in a posterior position, which often means a backache labour. Hilary says it felt like her back was going to break in two:

> Her back was to my back. I got down down all fours. I didn't want anyone to touch me. I spent the rest of the labour walking. At half past twelve, he asked me, 'Do you feel like pushing?' so I moved up in the bed. I was half sitting up. I was pushing for a hour. Even with all the people there, nobody could tell me how to push. I just couldn't get it. So he said to me, 'Do you want a bit of help?' I didn't know this meant a forceps and an episiotomy. I would have liked him to explain. So I had forceps, and an episiotomy, and I tore as well. I don't know how many stitches I had, but it was a lot.

'All the people' included two midwives, an obstetrician, several female friends and her husband. The forceps delivery left Hilary with a sense of failure. She put it down to not doing the 'right' things during labour, not resting, not eating, not urinating and being in the wrong delivery position.

Máire attributes her forceps delivery, the only other one in the group, to something else entirely:

> After they went downstairs to make tea, I could hear them saying, 'She's giving herself a good dose of it now.' I just wasn't there at all with the gas. I don't know what happened, but it just wasn't going to come out. I'd been pushing for an hour and a half. I was very nervous. They said there was some blood going down his throat.

Máire found the birth frightening: the baby was fine. She had been inhaling gas for two hours.

Margaret was hardly over the shock of discovering that the baby was breech when

> Gráinne said there was another baby. She was completely covered in the sac. Hannah didn't breathe. Gráinne gave her the kiss of life, and she was okay after a minute.

161

I got a terrible fright – I thought she was dead.

There was a second baby in there, another breech, and it was Hannah, the second twin, who showed up in the sample. Neither the breech, nor the twins, had been diagnosed. Many midwives feel detecting a breech should be possible, but with twins, it is difficult to distinguish one heartbeat from another. Both babies were fine.

In the group, one baby was born face sideways. A couple of babies emerged not only head first, but with a hand or an arm as well. 'He came out with his arm like this,' Leslie says, extending her arm fully, and nestling her head on top of it. The birth, she adds, was very quick, but very painful and tough. Leslie was unscathed, physically, unlike Sue, who tore badly: 'Her whole body just burst out. . . Her hand came with her head. My midwife said that was why I tore so badly.' She had what is known as a 'second degree' tear, extending into the muscles of the pelvic floor.

Sinéad's birth, her second, was one of the most demanding of all, physically:

The baby got stuck coming out. They were all shouting at me to push. I was pushing as hard as I could. She was stuck for about forty-five minutes. They were getting a bit panicky. I had to have an episiotomy in the end. The head stuck – she came out like this, with the forehead first. It was painful, very painful.

Her baby was positioned in what is known as a 'brow presentation', where the measurements of the head are at their widest. In hospital, a baby in this position is often delivered by Caesarian section. Sinéad was pushing for two hours: 'They couldn't do anything. I just had to get her out myself,' she says.

ॐ

Minutes and Hours

How long does it take for a baby to come out? For many women, this stage of labour – dreaded so much by so many – only lasts for a few minutes. Within the group, the average was 21 minutes. Mary Ellen was way over the average:

> I must have been pushing for at least an hour, fully dilated, with nothing happening. In the end I was worried about the oxygen, about brain damage.

She had a two-hour second stage, having been threatened with a 'high' forceps by the midwives at the antenatal clinic because of her 'poor muscle tone', her age (31) and the fact that she was having her fourth baby.

For the vast majority – 83 per cent – giving birth took less than half an hour. Of the remainder, ten women were pushing for an hour or more. Aylish, a former midwife, says it was at this point that she discovered why most women scream:

> They checked the fetal heart throughout and it was fine. They were so relaxed about it. There wasn't this wild panic to get the baby out. When he was born, I had an intact perineum. He was fine, very alert. In hospital, you get an hour, maybe two, at the most, if you're lucky.

An anterior lip on her cervix held up her labour. At just over four hours, she was pushing for longer than anyone else. Despite this, she sees it as a good birth, seeing herself as having been allowed to push the baby out herself, without the 'assistance' of a forceps.[49]

࿇

More Complications

Complications during this second stage were few and far between. Despite all the dire predictions women were often forced to listen to during pregnancy, 96 per cent of them had a perfectly normal birth.

Dympna's baby had a hard time:

I was pushing for two hours. But I was probably too tired. The head got slightly stuck, it came down and went up twice. Ten minutes before the end Louise listened to the baby's heart and it was getting weaker. 'You've got to get that baby out now,' she said to me. He was stressed. He was a bit bruised on his face, and he didn't suck for eight hours. He was a bit shaky and he had a wobbly chin.

Cord problems are something many women have heard of. Like haemorrhaging, they have assumed an almost mythical status in some women's minds, the stuff that nightmares are made of. One woman said the cord was tightly around the baby's neck, but she did not know if it was knotted, and she was not sure if it had been cut during delivery.

Another woman's contractions slowed down altogether during the second stage.

Once she saw the midwife sending for the doctor, Philomena says, she knew it was out of the usual routine:

There was blood whenever the pressure came. They wanted me to go to hospital. They were afraid the child would be exhausted. I was fine. It wasn't moving. I just wasn't making progress. The nurse said it was the muscles that were worn out. There was blood through the push. They were afraid the afterbirth was in the way, but it wasn't.

She was having her eighth baby at the age of 37.

Monica got a pain in her left leg during labour. Keeping it straight, she says, helped.

> I was fully dilated and the head wasn't coming down. The midwife sent for the doctor and he said if I couldn't get the head out, he'd use a forceps. The doctor went then. I just kept pushing. I got up to go to the toilet, and after that it was a flash of lightning. It's a terrific sensation once the head comes out. I couldn't get over how fat she was.

At 13lb, her baby weighed more than anyone else's. Asked how she felt when she realized she was in labour, she said it was no big deal. She was having her seventh child at home, breaking all the rules. At 44 years of age, Monica is the oldest woman in the group, and at 4ft 11in, the smallest in stature. Doctors would have regarded her as a miracle. Shoulder dystocia, they would say, with the baby stuck in transit, is the very least that could be expected.

꒰

Tearing

> I was in another world. There was a lot of force. It felt like I was going to split open [Máire].

Splitting open is a horrific prospect. Aylish says she had hoped to have an intact perineum. Many women were hoping to avoid an episiotomy. Having your perineum (the support structure of the pelvic floor) intact after birth also depends on not tearing. Over half, or 57 per cent, of the group came through completely unscathed, and a few others were very slightly grazed. The remainder were less fortunate, and although it was not often serious, 28 per cent of women tore. Midwives regard an intact perineum as an index of their professional skills, and these rates are in line with those published for home birth practices in the United States and in Britain.[50] Only nine per cent of the group were having their first babies, and the chances of coming through unscathed on a subsequent birth are greater.

A small tear is preferable to an episiotomy, women say. Only nine per cent had an episiotomy. Hilary was doubly disappointed; she tore after having had an episiotomy, but this is not uncommon.

Tears, like burns, are measured according to the severity of the injury sustained. A first degree tear is superficial. Midwives will tell you that a small tear causes less discomfort, and heals more quickly, if it is left to heal by itself, without being stitched. However, of the 21 per cent who suffered first degree tears, nearly everyone got stitched. Second degree tears, extending into the muscle, are a bit more serious, and five per cent of women suffered a tear of this magnitude.

Jo, the only one to suffer a third degree tear, had to go to hospital for a repair. Third degree tears extend as far as the rectum. Irish midwives do not usually do stitching at home. Carmel relates how they had to send for a doctor to do the suturing:

It was awful. He came in, and said we were lucky to have him, because he was working in the Iveagh at the time, and knew how to do the job. He had a terrible attitude, like he was coming in to some bizarre scene in the nineteenth century, being asked to stitch a woman who had just had a baby.

🙡

Delivering the Afterbirth

After the birth of a baby, the arrival of the afterbirth pales into insignificance. Many women hardly notice it coming, so taken up are they with the wonders of this just born baby. However, Sue, after a difficult birth, found it uplifting:

The midwife told me to stand up and the placenta was born – that was a pleasant experience. I felt my body had been splitting, but the placenta delivery was great.

Some women were hardly conscious of delivering the afterbirth as a separate entity. They just knew it must have slipped out, somehow. Midwives prefer the placenta to arrive fairly quickly, because there is a very slight risk that a woman may haemorrhage, and within the group, 19 minutes was the average. Mary describes how her placenta was a bit slow to arrive:

They said if it had been another 15 minutes, I'd have had to go to hospital. It was beautiful to see the placenta when it came out, to see what had kept her alive.

As many as 85 per cent of women delivered the afterbirth in less than 30 minutes, and 3 per cent took an hour or more.

From a clinical point of view, what is called the third stage of labour does not come to an end until whatever bleeding there is after the birth is under control. Only five per cent of women reported getting drugs to control bleeding such as ergometrine or syntometrine. But then, women do not necessarily remember whether or not they got an injection just as the baby's shoulder was being born, or indeed, immediately after the birth.[51] Not every midwife believes these drugs should be used routinely. And there may be less need for them when the afterbirth is allowed to deliver itself, without any of the pushing or the pulling associated with the active management of this stage of labour.[52]

Several women used a homeopathic equivalent of ergometrine, usually shepherd's purse. Thea, from an extensive stock of remedies, also used ladies' mantel 'to tone the uterus afterwards'.

Mary describes the last physical link between mother and child: 'The strength of the cord! It was pulsating violently. It was really fabulous to see it.' In most cases, the cord was cut only after it had stopped pulsating. Her husband was a bit nervous cutting the cord, Mary says, 'but he was proud at the same time'.

Cutting the cord is something men are occasionally asked to do. More often, they find themselves boiling water, having been dispatched by the midwife to get some. Boiling water has become part of the folklore surrounding home birth. Cecilia says you only need a small drop, just to sterilize the scissors for cutting the cord: 'I always thought you needed gallons of it,' she remarked.

At home, there was no tendency to hurry things. Professional time did not seem to matter in the same way. Niamh says her family doctor stayed for two or three hours after the birth: 'He seemed to be as happy as we were.' A bottle of wine might be opened, or some tea made and the entire family, the midwife, the doctor and whoever else was there, would sit around celebrating the arrival of a beautiful baby.

꒦

The Final Complications

One of the fears women have is the fear of haemorrhaging. Aylish points out that if you get a really massive haemorrhage, no matter where you are, you are finished: 'There's nothing they can do.' It is normal to lose some blood after giving birth. But how much is normal? Cecily Begley, an Irish midwife, suggests that women are well prepared during pregnancy for losing blood after birth. Losing between half and three-quarters of a pint is not a problem, she says, for healthy women.[53] Medically, losing more than half a pint is defined as a (postpartum) haemorrhage.

In the hours or days following birth (see Chapter 6), four women haemorrhaged, and three had what is known as 'retained secondary products', where the afterbirth does not come away cleanly. This is potentially risky as it could cause bleeding, and, in one case, it did. Altogether, five per cent of women had complications after delivery.

We expect women choosing home birth to want their husbands to be involved. We expect them to have clear preferences about birth, to be anti-pethidine, for example. We expect them to know their midwives. And we assume that they are all what obstetricians call 'low-risk'. This is the theory of home birth. Real life is different.

Everyone in the group obviously lived to tell the tale. In Western European countries, maternal mortality is almost a thing of the past. Infant mortality, however, is not. Within the group there were no dead babies, despite all the pessimistic predictions. Home birth studies around the world give perinatal mortality rates ranging from one to six per thousand births.[54] Maybe the group is not big enough. If three babies in every thousand die, that's only 0.3 in every hundred. In a group of 138, no deaths would be expected. However, the group is more like a typical hospital birth group than a typical home birth group.[55] Seven per cent of women would be classified by obstetricians as high risk.[56] This changes things. If 12 babies in every thousand die, nationally, in Ireland,[57] that is 1.2 babies in every hundred. Statistically, a death would not have been out of the question.

Home birth gives us a picture of birth without the machinery. A study like this can tell us how long labour can be expected to last in what women regard as a low-stress environment, unhurried by either drugs or instruments. It shows us how women meet the challenge of labour without resorting to painkillers. At home, each labour is a one-off, an original script. The study shows us how women, left to their own devices, prefer to write it. Above all, it shows us that labour is not necessarily synonymous with pain, any more than home birth is synonymous with danger.

Cradle and All

She bathed her, and put her on the kitchen scales. She toppled off twice, so they didn't do it again! Then I started getting cold. I went into my own room. There was an electric blanket on, it was lovely and warm. The only thing I didn't like was Mary [the midwife] rubbing her hard with an old towel, which had been lying at the bottom of the bed. I'd had the softest towel . . . I sat bolt upright in bed. Kieran had been dancing around the place with her, laughing and crying. She yanked her out of Kieran's hands, and started rubbing her. I suppose it was good for the circulation . . . It was great to be able to get into your own bed, and have your husband there beside you, a nice warm body! [Christina]

The first days and weeks after birth are crucial. They can also be difficult. At home there may not be the luxury of a breathing-space. Those few days where everything is done for you depend on others, those days when you can lie back and accept the congratulations, the flowers, and the good wishes of family and friends.

It is a demanding time, a time for being looked after, for help with the baby, for help in the house. Postnatal visits do not always materialize. Some women were expected to get up the next day to cook the dinner. Establishing a routine with a new baby while at the same time trying to get yourself back to normal is not easy. Breast-feeding can bring its own difficulties. Euphoric, chaotic, intense and exhausting is how a Dutch psychologist, Ingerlise Andersen, describes this period.[1] For a small number of women, it all proved too much. They got depressed. Hardly any of them got help.

॰ॐ

At the Summit

There was no sense of ice. I felt I'd lost nothing as a woman by it.
Total joy, elation, relief. It was wonderful! I was happy!
We dreamed of heaven that night.

Katherina's partner told her to open her eyes to see the baby:

There was such a huge distance between before the birth and after it. Although it was maybe only a second, I don't know, it was as if I were in the cosmos, coming back from eternity, to see the baby.

Nora also talks about 'coming down' from 'another world', about the 'unreality' of it all. For three-quarters of the group, those first moments after birth were exhilarating. Thrilled, delighted, elated, amazed, these are the words they use. Some women believe you can only feel like this if you do not have drugs, as Claire, a nurse, explains:

I was thrilled, elated, absolutely excited, something I didn't experience on Roberta because I was too drugged. This dampens down your natural elation after giving birth.

Knowing that she did it without 'anything' gave her an added buzz, Lorna recalls: 'Afterwards, it was terribly exhilarating, to have done it with no mind-altering drugs.'
Noelle, a former midwife, only felt a sense of relief: 'I was

half stupid! I didn't give a damn! Pure relief, that he was born, that he was okay, that I was okay.' It is a time when waves of emotions come flooding in, one after another. Relief can become joy. Máire, after a forceps delivery, felt glad to be alive: 'The birds were singing, and the sun was shining, and I was glad to be at home.' Not everyone was so lucky. Jacintha describes how she just wanted everyone to go away:

> I felt low. I felt I was in a deep pit. I was excited, numb. Playing to the gallery. It was a type of depression, like there was someone else performing. I thought 'I can't spoil it for them.'

Sometimes, there is an anxiety to return to normal life, a sense of wanting to be released from the top of the mountain. A few women were shocked. Lucinda says it was as though someone had given her a letter:

> The effect of coming down off that was powerful. I was terribly shocked. I felt disappointed. I had no sense of elation.

When Emily got over the shock, she was furious. She felt like she had been conned into training for a marathon, only to find herself in an egg-and-spoon race:

> For about twenty minutes I was very disappointed. Where was all that puffing and panting you read about in the books? Six, seven or eight hours in labour? . . . I was angry, yes. All those books on childbirth, all written by bloody men. They haven't got a clue.

She had a one-hour labour.

❧

First View

The midwife pushed me on to the bed. 'It's a boy!' she said, thinking the cord was . . . She must have got a fright. She was gorgeous! She was tiny and she had these enormous eyes [Denise].

I got him first. He came out gleaming, spotless. I'd never seen a spotless baby before [Nuala].

He was like an albino. He was very fair, with very fair lashes. He looked just like a peach. He was plump looking, a beautiful baby, with that furry hair [Gina].

She roared, poohed and weed all over the carpet! . . . Catherine was two years and two months at the time. She came to the door and said, 'Daddy – baby – Waaagh'! [Susan]

I didn't like her at all. I don't like new babies. I knew she wouldn't look like the baby on the Pampers' box. Those yucky, bluey things covered in gunk are beautiful? They're not really nice until they're six months old [Emily].

'She was extremely beautiful', Ute says, 'the complete miracle of life! Touchable!' However, not every woman feels an instant rush of love for this baby who is so suddenly *there*. Ursula puts it down to being in a daze:

He had my husband's nose! I was dazed, not particularly overjoyed, a bit detached. By the next morning I was in love with him.

Irene says she was so tired and sore that she did not want to see her son. She told the midwife to take him away. How you feel about the baby can depend on how you feel yourself.

Christina admits to 'slight' disappointment that it was not a boy: 'I never thought I'd feel that. But it was very fleeting.' A few women remark on how delighted they were to discover that it was a boy – or a girl. Gender matters in our society.

Looking at the baby can mean looking at the midwife handling the baby:

> She was mucousy. I watched her changing colour. She was a bit blue, in her arms and legs. For about thirty seconds, we just waited for her to cry. She whacked her. She just held her upside down by the ankles and she slapped her. She could have done it more gently. Naturally she screamed [Lelia].

The previous generation of babies were often slapped to get them to cry: crying was regarded as good for the lungs. It is a long way from a Leboyer birth, which is what Lelia wanted. This entails immersing the baby in warm water as soon as possible after the birth, to recreate the watery element from which she has just come. Enya describes the result:

> He was placed on the breast for a little while, and then into water. He completely unfolded, bloomed like a little flower and smiled.

Holding the baby immediately, putting her to the breast, this is how many women wanted it. 'It's not just the birth, it's afterwards,' says Ursula. Four-fifths of the group held their babies immediately after they were born. Betty says she held her son while the midwife was still fixing her up:

> After, she wrapped him and put him in his cot while the doctor was stitching me. She waited until I was nice and comfortable before giving him to me again. She put mother first! Once you get a cup of tea and a cigarette, you come back to life.

༂

Birthweight

Having absorbed the fact that it is a girl, or a boy, the next thing many women want to know is what weight the baby is. Since the beginning of the century, when regular weighing of newborn babies was introduced, birthweight has come to signify health.[2] Three-quarters of the babies weighed from over three to four and a half kilos, or over six and a half to ten pounds approximately. Peggy was anxious for the doctor to leave in case he might 'cop on'. She had a small 'small' baby:

> I wrapped her in four blankets. She weighed four pounds, but she wasn't even three and a half, I'd say, with all those blankets.

When it comes to labour outcomes, birthweight is regarded by doctors as one of the critical factors, like gestation. It was a Finnish doctor working in Germany in the 1920s who observed that being born too small was different from being born too early; he suggested 2,500g, five and a half pounds, as the limit, and this is still used today to define 'small' babies.[3] Low birthweight is associated with increased risks of death, illness and disability.[4] Peggy says she would prefer to have them small: 'When they're small, you have to love them all the time.'

The smallest of all the small babies belongs to Rita, who had a lump removed from her breast during pregnancy. She had a five-minute labour; her daughter weighed three pounds at birth. Several of her babies had been small when they were born, but this child was the smallest.

Within the group, six per cent of the babies were small. This is high for a home birth group, and it probably reflects the fact that the group includes a small number of women who would be classified by doctors as high-risk. Fewer small babies are born at home;[5] women having home births tend to be better

175

off, and therefore healthier. When small babies are born at home, however, they may do better. British researcher Rona Campbell, in her study of home births in England and Wales, showed that the perinatal mortality rate for small babies born at home was considerably less than the national rate for babies of the same weight.[6]

None of the small babies were premature, none of them were admitted to hospital after the birth, and their mothers reported no problems with them, apart from the extra minding they entailed. Peggy, a mother of five children, says this baby was the only one she attempted to breastfeed. She started her on spoon feeds at three weeks:

> The doctor was mesmerized. He said, 'Her stomach isn't big enough to take that.' When he came back and saw her a few weeks later, he said, 'Fair play!'

There were some huge babies. Nine per cent weighed over four and a half kilos, or over ten pounds. Niamh's baby weighed ten pounds two ounces: 'When I saw her, I thought where in the name of God had I put her? She looked enormous, massive.' She was not the top of the range. The record for heavyweight babies within the group was held by Monica's baby, who weighed in at thirteen pounds.

Complications After Delivery

Five women had to go to hospital for complications after the birth. Jo went in, together with her baby (who had jaundice), to have a third-degree tear repaired:

> During the night, I had an overwhelming desire to grab him and run. I felt very primeval – just like animals are. They never brought him to me for feeding.

The nurses were very nice, she says, but 'the doctor treated me as an irresponsible crank, a hippy type'.

Both Ingrid and Cindy had to have medical treatment following an unattended birth (see Chapter 7). Ingrid haemorrhaged within hours after the birth, and was given two blood transfusions in hospital. The day after the birth, Cindy went in to have a small tear on a vein repaired, only to be told that there was a bit of the afterbirth still inside. She had to have a D & C (dilatation and curettage of the womb), to remove 'secondary products' said to have been retained after the birth. So did another woman who haemorrhaged. Cora relates how she felt okay for the first week. Then she had a bleeding, got sent to hospital, and was given a blood transfusion. The bleeding, she was told, was due to an infection.

Altogether, three per cent of women haemorrhaged within the group, and this is in line with rates quoted for home birth elsewhere.[7]

⁂

Getting Up

Lesley got up an hour after the birth. It was Christmas Eve, and her husband was having trouble wrapping the children's presents. Connie says, with pride, that she got up after two hours. Ute was up bringing in turf for the fire three hours later: 'I didn't rest.' This determination to carry on as usual, this refusal to rest, can come from very different sources. For Ute, it is a statement about how 'natural' birth is to women: 'Tribeswomen and nomads carry on working,' she says. Connie was simply determined not to let the birth interfere with her life, any more than she would allow child-bearing to affect her figure. Other women stayed in bed for a week.

Depending on who is doing the cooking and the washing, getting up may also depend on feeling well. Not many women had health problems, and 73 per cent had not got a single complaint. Christina talks about the luxury of being able to take a shower: 'I got up the next morning and had a shower – you wouldn't be allowed to do that in hospital.' Some women make similar comments.

Monica, who had had a pain in her leg during labour, developed a clot: 'The doctor put me on medication and it cleared up within a week.' Looked at medically, hers was the most potentially serious health complaint. Four women got a vaginal infection, such as thrush, and two got a kidney infection. Several women developed mastitis, and another woman got a chest infection. One woman developed phlebitis, an inflammation of the veins.

Not being sick does not necessarily mean feeling good. However, some women were of the opinion that because of the unbroken continuity and the calmness of home, you don't get the blues. The night her son was born, Deirdre says, echoing the words of other women, it was as if he had always been there:

> I got up the next day. There was no break like there is when you go to hospital. You are pampered. Everything is done for you, then you go home.

Miriam, another nurse, feels that at home, you do not have the same doubts about your ability to manage the baby: 'There was no let-down afterwards, no change of environment, no anxiety.' Researchers have suggested that women rarely suffer from 'baby blues' at home,[8] but the study shows otherwise. By far the largest number of problems women report in the days following birth are to do with emotional well-being. Eight per cent of women suffered from baby blues. Sometimes known as 'third' or 'fourth' day blues, this is when women are most likely to feel low, when they experience mood swings or have bouts of crying for 'no reason', as Ann Oakley has pointed out.[9] In her study, 84 per cent of women suffered from baby blues. Within this group, some women also suffered from more serious depression.

ॐ

Putting the Food on the Table

I took charge immediately. My mother couldn't believe it.
She stayed in bed for most of a week at home after her
babies were born [Maeve].

If everything is done for you in hospital, how much is done for
you at home, and for how long? Within the group, lack of help
at home during those first, demanding days is a universal
complaint. It is the main disadvantage of having a home birth,
as far as a lot of women are concerned. So it was for Amanda,
living with her family in a mobile home on the edge of a lake:

I didn't have any help at all. I was on my own for the first
week after the birth. My husband was working. I found it
very difficult. Having no help in the house is the big disadvantage of having a home birth.

During the first 10 days, fathers helped to varying degrees.
Some did everything. Others did nothing, and 10 per cent of
women had to manage on their own. Máire tells of how she
had to make tea for herself, even though she could hardly
walk, after a forceps delivery:

After he was born, I got up. There was no one there. My
husband was asleep. I went downstairs on my bottom to
make tea. Then I went back to bed for the day. I got up
after that – the food had to be put on the table.

Máire felt she had no choice about putting the food on the
table. At home, according to Linda, life goes on as usual:

It's like Christmas, only much better. You've got this
wonderful present. It was lovely. I was up by midday the
next day, and I prepared the evening meal.

A third of the group drafted in family and friends to help. Neighbours would take the kids, Betty explains. 'If you came in, you were volunteered! I spent the whole week in bed.' But such arrangements tended to be sporadic, fragmented and unpredictable. Lelia was lucky – her mother came in and helped: 'She looked after the two children, and did the cooking for about two weeks. And I had Sean for a week.' Frequently, only paid help could be seen to offer the kind of organized, structured and reliable support that women need at this critical time. But although more women could, in theory at least, have afforded to pay someone to come in, only seven per cent did so.

Beatrix feels it was a bit rough not having any support: 'House help should be available'. Beatrix is Dutch; in Holland a maternity nurse's aide comes in for eight days after the birth.[10] She does everything that needs to be done, from helping with breast-feeding to doing the washing and the cooking. However, keeping an eye on mother and baby is regarded as one of her more important functions. Having a home birth in Ireland is another story. Harriet sums it up: 'Life does tend to require you to get up the next day.' In theory, local health boards can provide women with a home help service after birth, but this is not something that is generally known. Only three women, one of whom was Margaret, who gave birth to twins, got a home help from the state at this time.

༄

Well Babies

She didn't cry till she was two weeks old. We phoned the doctor. He laughed. He said, 'You mean to say she hasn't cried till now?' [Emily].

Nearly every baby was a well baby, and 91 per cent of women had no difficulties whatsoever with their babies during the first month. Not gaining weight was the most common problem: Women have been taught to regard regular weight gain as a sign of good health in babies.[11]

The twins were among the few babies who had problems. They were admitted to hospital during the first week: Morgon was sent in on the fourth day with a suspected kidney infection, and Hannah went in two days later with anaemia. They both received blood transfusions, and these were repeated a few weeks later. Another baby to be admitted to hospital was Jo's. Jo is Rhesus Negative, she had developed antibodies which had passed through the placenta to her baby, causing him to break down his blood cells and, as a result, become jaundiced. He was the second baby in the group to be admitted to hospital for jaundice. He was kept in for two days, under the lights, for phototherapy.

Thirty-six hours after the birth, Deborah, a nurse, started to get worried about her baby daughter: 'She would go blue for a minute, and then her colour would come back.' She brought her to the out-patients' department. The staff thought she was a Caesarian section – her head was perfectly round – and they identified the cause of the 'blueness':

> I delivered her in a very upright position, sitting on the edge of an armchair. So on the way out, she got an extra transfusion of blood from the placenta, and it was the extra haemoglobin that was making her blue.

They said she was very healthy, and that it was a good sign.

Several other babies had problems. One baby developed a chest infection, another got an ear infection, and a third got a 'strep' (a streptococcal bacterial) umbilical infection. Dympna's baby was left with a chin wobble after a tough birth, but it disappeared at five months.

Looking at who was hospitalized, and why, is one way doctors measure health among newborn babies born at home.[12] If we include Deborah's daughter, who was seen as an outpatient, we get a hospitalization rate for babies of three per cent, and this is identical to national rates quoted for Dutch babies born at home.[13] Unfortunately, these rates in the group are slightly lower than they might have been. Other babies who might have been admitted to hospital, were not. Congenital defects were not always picked up.

Another way of measuring health among full-term babies which is used by doctors is to look at the incidence of convulsions during the first 48 hours of life.[14] None of the babies in the group had convulsions. If you want to measure 'morbidity', if you want to rule out the possibility of damage to a baby during birth, it makes sense to look at a child's long-term development. Jane describes how her son was slow to talk, adding that he is fine now. No one else within the group reported that there had been a problem with their children's development.

৵

Hungry Babies

The vast majority of the group chose to breast-feed their babies. Home birth mothers tend to breast-feed.[15] Only one-sixth of the group, usually women who were less well-off, bottle-fed their babies. It is mainly middle-class women who breast-feed nowadays, Maeve believes, underlining the shift in social attitudes since the 1950s:

> My mother breast-fed us, and in those times, nobody breast-fed unless they couldn't afford the bottles.

Three-quarters of the mothers breast-fed for at least six months, while almost a third continued for over a year. This is much higher than average for Ireland, where only a third of women breast-feed initially, and only two-thirds of these are still breast-feeding six weeks after the birth.[16] It is a bottle-feeding culture, as Efa shows:

> I knew nothing about babies. I didn't even know what

SMA [a formula milk] was. One day in the salon, when I was pregnant, a woman asked me what milk would I give her, and I said 'Well, I suppose, Premier or Avonmore, [bottled milk]. And the woman laughed.

Six women changed over to bottle-feeding during the first four weeks:

I'd bottle-fed the others, and thought I'd try breast-feeding. I did it for two days, but I felt embarrassed in front of the children. The nurse called once a day.

It was Ellen's sixth baby, and it was her first attempt to breast-feed. She felt she needed more support.

Cassie also breast-fed for two days but she got sore nipples. As many as seven per cent of women had physical difficulties with breast-feeding, suffering from cracked nipples, breast abscesses or infections. It was the single biggest problem area for women in terms of their physical health. Cassie was told by her doctor that the baby was not getting enough milk, and that she would have to switch to bottles. She did not have a single visit from a midwife or a public health nurse. Women complain about lack of support from staff in hospital, about the difficulties created by scheduled feeding and restricted access to the baby (see Chapter 2). At home, lack of hands-on advice and support is also identified as one of the main difficulties, particularly during those first days.

ॐ

Health Visitors

At home they weren't racing off. They had time to sit and talk to you. There was no one rushing you [Niamh].

As well as help in the house and help with breast-feeding,

women may need help with 'after' pains and with caring for a new baby. Like 'house' help during the first ten days, postnatal care was conspicuous by its absence. Women were often left to fend for themselves. Some women only got one or two visits from their midwives. A few never saw their midwives again after the birth, while others did not see their doctors.

There was a huge variation in the number of visits women received from their midwives after the birth. At the top end of the scale, eight per cent of women were visited more than once a day, for 10 days by their midwife. Older, district midwives tended to visit their clients more often than younger, independent midwives. If you took the view that one or two visits, or none, simply was not enough, then 12 per cent of women had inadequate care. And if you took the view that a minimum of seven visits over ten days amounted to 'good' care, then only 39 per cent of women got that level of attention.

Another official health visitor is the public health nurse. In an unattended birth, the public health nurse will be the only health visitor. Only a third of the group were visited by a public health nurse during the first 10 days after the birth.

No one complained about lack of postnatal care, however. Perhaps women did not know that they were entitled to daily visits for up to fourteen consecutive days from their midwives. This used to be the standard, but now there are no standards, because, officially, there are no home births. Perhaps they did not know that they were also entitled to a visit from a public health nurse, and that looking after mothers and babies is, officially, part of public health nursing.[17]

Overall, this lack of support has all kinds of implications. Mothers of small babies got less than adequate care during the first 10 days. Of the six mothers who gave up breast-feeding early, five were visited infrequently, or not at all, by their midwives. Finally, some babies born with congenital problems went undiagnosed for weeks or months, and for one child, this had serious, long-term consequences.

୬

Testing For PKU

I wouldn't let her [the public health nurse] do the heel test. She said it was to see if she was absorbing nourishment. But anyone could see she was absorbing nourishment. She was feeding and putting on weight. The only reason for it that I could see was a bureaucratic reason. The nurse had to get her pink form filled in.

Grace was not going to let the nurse stick a needle in her baby, she says, just for the sake of a pink form. Six women refused to allow the test to be done.

The 'heel' or 'PKU' test is a national screening programme for newborn babies, diagnosing not only PKU, but other metabolic disorders. PKU, or phenylketonuria – more common in Ireland than in any other European country[18] – can cause irreversible brain damage but the progress of the disease can be retarded if the baby's diet is adjusted. Public health nurses did not always seem to be able to explain what the heel test was for:

The public health nurse wanted to do it [the PKU test] about four weeks later, but from what she said, it was mainly to find out about this disease which was hereditary, I think, and found mainly in the west [of Ireland].

Claudine, who is from Geneva, saw herself as being outside the genetic pool of the west of Ireland. In all, seven per cent of babies went untested. In the case of three of them, it was because the midwife or the doctor forgot to do it.

ᔓ

Feeling Depressed

Mona never told her husband or her family how she was feeling:

He was crying day and night. He even cried while he was being fed. Twenty minutes was the most he ever slept. I brought him to the doctor, and he said he had colic. I just knew he was a crying baby. I was very, very depressed. It was unbelievable, desperate. I started getting headaches – they thought I'd fluid in my ears. I was completely exhausted. I went to the doctor with tension headaches – he gave me Valium. People warned me against it, so I didn't bother to take them. I never went out – you wouldn't leave a crying baby like that to anyone. One daughter was great with him – but even she had to hand him back again. I had a pal, and we fell out. Everything fell apart. I'd be sitting there, and my eyes would fill up, and I'd want to cry. I got nervous. I felt sure something was going to happen to me. I used to wonder how I was going to get through the house[work]. It went, eventually. It took a few months.

Some women seem to think postnatal depression is unique to hospital birth. 'At home there's none of this drop-back effect,' says Biddy. Like other women, she feels that birth in hospital is hyped up to be a big performance that gets applause and flowers from the (visiting) audience. Then when it is all over, it is back home to the routine of real life. Within the group, nine per cent of women got depressed. They suffered from much more than a sense of anti-climax after the birth, or feelings of anxiety in relation to the baby.

In other studies, rates for postnatal depression from 8 to 25 per cent have been quoted.[19] These rates tend to be based on the experiences of women who delivered in hospital. It is not clear whether the place of birth has a bearing on postnatal depression but the link between postnatal depression and a technological experience of birth has been made.[20] Of the 11 women in the group who had had postnatal depression on a previous birth, 10 had experienced a traumatic hospital birth.

An Edinburgh-based psychologist, Carole Mhic Shíomóin, defined postnatal depression as referring to 'those kinds of depression which are mild enough to enable women to continue somehow, but severe enough to make them feel that life is pretty dreary and intolerable'.[21] Ute got depressed seven weeks after the birth. She explains it by saying, 'It was over-tiredness . . . In two and a quarter years, I slept one night.' Her partner was in and out of work. She relates how when he was unemployed, he used to drink, and when he was working, he was away from home. Not long after the birth, they split up. She got no help from anybody.

Postnatal depression usually lasts for months rather than weeks. It may peak during the first three months, but it can peak any time during the second half of the baby's first year.[22] Rita, who had a lumpectomy during pregnancy, says her nerves went when her daughter was 12 months. Since then she has been attending an out-patients' psychiatric clinic. She has had the lymph nodes under her arm removed; doctors have told her that it is not cancer.

Within the group, postnatal depression went largely unrecognized and untreated. Six women suffering from depression endured it for 12 months or more. Both Mona and Ute went to their family doctor, to no apparent avail. Others, like Jo and Carmel, did not consult a professional at all. Jo saw her depression as resulting from the enforced separation from her baby, who was hospitalized for jaundice shortly after birth. Carmel blamed her mother-in-law: 'She was going through a nervous breakdown at the time – I was like a sitting duck for her to unload.'

Rose is the only one who was hospitalized. She had a history of depression. A few weeks after her baby was born, she became depressed again. In hospital and separated from her baby, she was treated with electro-convulsive therapy and drugs: 'It didn't take away from the birth,' she says. 'The birth was wonderful.' Overtiredness, crying babies, nervy mothers-in-law, absent partners, isolation, lack of support, these are some of the explanations women give for feeling depressed.[23] Rose is the only one to see her depression in a wider context: 'There were a lot of things going on in my life at the time. My mother died a few months before the birth.'

Emily says she felt great up to a month after her baby was born:

By the time she was four months, I'd gone to thirteen stone. I was a foodaholic. I never ate in public. I used to hide food all over the house. I went to the doctor. He said I was just a hysterical woman. I got no help from anyone. My husband was away all the time. It was easy to put on a show at weekends. I remember once, when she was five months, taking her lock, stock and barrel, buggy, nappies, the lot, to his office. I handed her to him and said, 'Here,' turned on my heel and walked out the door. He had nothing to feed her with. His boss said to him: 'Your wife is suffering from postnatal depression.' And he said: 'There's nothing the matter with her.'

Several women who suffered from depression had poor or difficult family relationships, particularly with their mothers. Emily was seven when her parents divorced. She came home from boarding-school at Easter to find her mother was no longer there. Her postnatal depression lasted for three years. None of her children have 'ever' slept. She says that she suffers from agoraphobia, a fear of open or public spaces, and marriage: 'I hate being married.'

⌇

Imperfect Babies

Discovering that your perfect baby is imperfect can be a shock. And when you have nursed him for weeks, or even for months, not knowing there is anything the matter, then the shock must be all the greater. Vicki, who received just one or two visits from her midwife after the birth, says her son was checked over only when he was born:

> But she didn't check him after that, just his belly button. He wasn't pissing properly. You know the way little boys piss, straight up? He was just dribbling ... At five weeks I went to the doctor to register him. He seemed to be getting worse. The doctor said to bring him to the hospital. I mentioned to one of the nurses that he wasn't peeing properly. They thought I wasn't feeding him properly, that he wasn't getting enough milk. They had him on a drip for two days. You could see him swelling up. His bladder became so swollen, it was completely blocked. He vomited blood. I had a row with the doctor. He was transferred to another hospital. They wouldn't let us go in the ambulance with him. He was very, very, very ill. There was a valve blocked in his penis.

He was in hospital for five months. Afterwards, he got one infection after another. According to his mother, one kidney is gone and only a third of the other is functioning. When he is eighteen, she says, he will have to have dialysis, and a kidney transplant.

Vicki thought of bringing a court case against the first hospital, where his kidneys got 'flooded':

> But a consultant told me it could get very vicious, the fact that I'd had a home birth, that I wasn't married, that the case against the hospital would be very difficult to prove. He asked me if I could take the strain, and I said I didn't know.

She dropped the idea of litigation. With hindsight, she feels that had he been born in a hospital, his condition would probably have been noticed, but it is very rare, she emphasizes. Had she been listened to by hospital staff, or had she been visited more frequently by her midwife, the outcome might have been different.

ᴖ

Rachel's Story

My mother said she wasn't thriving. That was the first time anyone had said that. I had to wean her at five months. She got a bit of a cold. She started vomiting . . . The doctor said she had whooping cough . . . I noticed that her lips were slightly blue. She was a week less than seven months when I decided to bring her to another doctor. He said, 'Her lips are slightly blue.' I couldn't see it. He brought her outside, and I still couldn't see it. He told me to bring her in straightaway. She had congestive heart failure.

She was a hole-in-the-heart baby with multiple problems. Had she lived, her mother was told, she would have needed a heart and lung transplant. Rachel remembers how neighbours said things like, 'What can you expect?' as she had been born at home:

But the professor said there were two factors which contributed to the fact that she had lived till then. One was the breast-feeding, the other was the fact that she had been born at home. If she'd been born in hospital, she might have picked up an infection . . . I was glad I had that seven months with her, not knowing.

She was seven months old when she died. As Barbara Katz Rothman so clearly shows in her book on prenatal diagnosis, foreknowledge can make the future intolerable.[24]

Elizabeth's son was five months old before she discovered that he had a heart condition, a valve problem, but she expects him to grow out of it without any need for surgery.

Babies are sometimes born with their hips out of alignment, and this is something midwives and doctors usually check. Noticed early on, the remedy is simple enough. At ten months however, it is too late for extra nappies or a splint for support, as Ger discovered: 'We only found out when he was ten months. He was put in plaster for three months, but he didn't need surgery.'

All of these problems were diagnosed late. Olive's son, born with a 'rockerbottom' foot, was the only baby whose problem did not go unnoticed; his difference was particularly visible:

In hospital, they said it was the way he was handled at birth. But I know myself it would have been the same if he'd been born in hospital. The doctor said it was the way he was lying in the womb.

Her son has been operated on twice.

At four per cent, the rate for congenital problems is higher than those quoted for other home birth groups.[25] Home birth mothers tend to be healthier than the general population, and their babies tend to have fewer congenital problems.

ॐ

Thinking Back Over It All

There is no comparison, women say, between birth at home and birth in hospital. No matter how efficient or caring they are in hospital, you are able to relax at home, they say, to do what you want. Women who choose to stay at home tend to be pleased with their experience of birth.[26] Margaret says she was delighted with her home birth. The fact that she had undiagnosed breech twins did not put her off: 'I don't think I could have a hospital delivery after it.' The majority of women – 71 per cent – were pleased with the way things had gone, while 14 per cent were displeased, and the remainder seemed to have no strong feelings one way or the other. Florence says the birth was exactly what she wanted: 'No technology, no noise, no strangers.'

For seven women, emotionally, the birth was a calamity. They use words like 'awful' to describe it, and in no circumstances would they repeat it. Their experience is worth looking at more closely. What they shared, apart from uncomplicated labours, was a lack of belief in themselves and in their ability to give birth. At the critical moment, they felt they just could not do it. Denise relied on pethidine to get her through. Máire, left alone by her midwife and doctor, nearly gassed herself (see Chapter 5). What they also shared was a poor relationship with the professional involved. Cora did not have a working relationship with her midwife, any more than Denise. She complained that the midwife did not want to touch her while she was in labour and that she hardly spoke to her.

Several women were left with a sense of damaged self-esteem. One of them is Mary Ellen, whose confidence had been well and truly shattered by hospital midwives during her pregnancy. At her age, and with her muscle tone, they said, she should not be having a home birth. The experience left her with a sense of personal failure, and a feeling that she had had a narrow escape: 'I felt I had just squeaked by.' She blames herself for the fact that she was pushing for two hours:

I should have done more walking, more swimming. I was just lazy. I should have been more physical. Maybe then I might have been a better pusher.

Feelings of anxiety, insecurity, lack of autonomy, lack of confidence, as well as lack of communication with one's midwife or doctor, these are the hallmarks of a 'bad' birth. Home birth is not for every woman, apparently.

Listening to women talking about their experiences at home, certain themes begin to emerge. Three-quarters of the group were pleased with their professional care. Charlotte says her midwife gave her a sense of competence: 'I didn't know her from Adam.' There was a feeling that, together, they had done a good job. Gina says her midwife was fabulous:

She was very confident and efficient, just completely professional. There was no fuss, but she was meticulous about everything. Everything would be sterile. She was very organized.

Many women feel a sense of gratitude to their midwives and to their doctors for giving them what they regard as crucial support at a stressful time. Nora sees this as the key difference between having a baby at home and having one in hospital. In hospital, she claims, drugs and intervention are a substitute for personal contact.

At home, intervention is part of what women are trying to avoid, and a number of women remark with satisfaction on how 'natural' the birth was. Irene does not believe in natural childbirth, but she appreciated the lack of interference: 'I was very pleased with the midwife. You weren't hassled, poked at or messed with.'

Only a small minority were dissatisfied with their midwives or doctors and invariably, relations between them were strained. As soon as the doctor came, Lucinda says, she slipped back into being 'a good little girl', for some unaccountable reason: 'He forced the pushing, but I wanted him to be there . . . I wasn't happy with him. He was too distant. He lacked sensitivity.'

Within the group, autonomy is always a major issue. At home, where there is no system to be resisted, the focus tends to be more on coping with the demands of labour. Women talk about feeling relaxed, confident and able to cope, instead of feeling afraid, tense or anxious. For many women, staying in control of themselves, and of their labour, is an achievement, a source of pride and satisfaction. Natural childbirth has taught women to value self control. Some women believe it is much easier to maintain control at home than it is in hospital.

Conversely, losing control of yourself in labour is regarded by many as one of the worst things that can happen. Helena felt that she had overreacted, that she had shouted too much. Ashling says she wanted to 'take it easy', but instead:

It was panic stations! I didn't handle it well. I was roaring.
Joe, my neighbour, could hear me. He was pacing up and
down. The whole street could hear me. I was mortified.

But she enjoyed the birth, despite having only her aunt, very
reluctantly, in attendance.

At home, autonomy can mean being able to go for a walk in
labour, or stay in the bath for hours. Some women were particularly pleased with the delivery position they adopted. A few,
like Aileen, regretted this feature of the birth:

I would have preferred not to be on my back. I felt that
might have been the reason for the episiotomy. I felt in
control when I was upright.

Unpicking the threads of autonomy from the tightly woven
fabric of women's stories, there is a feeling of being in control,
a sense of self-determination, which seemed to flow from
being at home. Many women feel it gave them the space
in which to decide things for themselves, and that they made
the most of it. 'I felt I had the baby myself,' Rosemary says,
summing up the feelings of three-quarters of the group. As
far as Ursula is concerned, autonomy comes with the territory:

At home I felt confident, secure, empowered. In hospital I
was totally submissive, passive, in the power of others . . .
At home I never stopped being myself. When I grazed
myself, I just shot up and screamed. I enjoyed letting rip,
having the privacy, the space to do it in.

Ursula was the only one who felt that she was entitled to let rip
when she was in labour, to behave as she did.

For a small minority of women, it is precisely this facet of
the birth that was unsatisfactory. Hilary is one of the few who
felt she did not do it herself, that she had a passive delivery
rather than an active birth:

It didn't live up to my idea of what it ought to be. I felt it

194

was taken away from me, that I didn't perform.

Her baby was posterior (see Chapter 5). She felt her birth was mismanaged, that she had not been given the support she needed, and that the forceps delivery could have been avoided. Just as when there is no established relationship with the midwife or doctor, lack of autonomy is a marker for a negative experience.

At home, a father can be anything from a minor acolyte, asked to boil water by the midwife, to the director of the movie. There are women who stress their partner's role in the birth, sometimes to the point of obscuring their own, but they are in a minority. Men's role was primarily to help women cope with the stress of labour. 'It was the fact that he was there, his physical presence. It was moral support,' Catherine says, speaking for two-thirds of the group. For most women, the fact that he was there was clearly a source of deep satisfaction. Statia compares it to crossing a stream with him halfway there:

> There are these stones. You're crossing a ford, and he's holding out his hand to you, and saying, 'You can do it.' You reach that wall in labour. You can be coaxed through it.

Frieda felt that her relationship with her husband improved as a result of his being present at the birth.

It did not always work out. A few felt their husbands were no help to them in labour. Jean's husband was in considerable distress: 'He had to be calmed by the midwife during the labour. He wasn't any good to me.' For a few others, the fact that, for one reason or another, their husbands were absent at the critical moment was a source of regret.

Women's stories about birth are about their relationships – with themselves, their partners, their midwives and doctors, and their babies. The idea of a gentle birth has become widespread. Sue explains her daughter's placid personality in terms of her birth: 'She is a very easy child. She had a good birth – no trauma, no drugs, no interference, no noise.' For Rachel, as for others, being left on her own with her daughter, after it was all over, was the best part of it: 'I remember it was snowy and crisp outside. I had some tea, then I snuggled down in bed with Ciara.'

Birth does not end with the cutting of the cord. For many women, being able to put the baby to the breast straightaway is part of it all. 'Bonding', in whatever guise, comes up again and again. Florence says she is much closer to her second daughter born at home than she is to her first daughter born in hospital: 'She's a little devil, but . . . I put it down to better bonding.' Whether in mother-child, father-child, or brother-and-sister relationships, women see bonding as something that flows from the physical proximity at birth and the unbroken continuity of home. The fact that their children were around, that they were able to bring them in to see the new baby within minutes or hours of the birth, to curl up in bed together, these are the things that matter. The children arrived as the baby was being born, Charlotte recalls: 'To hear them talking about it afterwards, it was normal. It was natural. It was a family thing.' Niamh's two-year-old thought the baby was a present: 'We have a photo of Deirdre on the bed with the baby, clapping her hands. She had had a birthday a few days before.'

Women value the privacy, intimacy and seclusion of home. It is something that those who have had a previous hospital birth tend to mention. Brenda states that the sheer peace and privacy of the birth was 'Indescribable. There was a sense of harmony and warmth.'

A small number of women were disappointed with long and difficult labours. A sixth of the group thought theirs bad enough to comment on. Ger describes her experience as 'Cruel. It was the worst birth possible.' Such vehemence was rare, however. Catherine had a 16-hour labour: 'The cord was round the neck. He was facing the wrong way.' The descent of this 11lb baby was slow and laboured. This is what Catherine had to say about it:

If the birth had been faster, I would have torn. If he'd come down quicker, he would have strangled on the cord.

I had two internals, one to see how things were, the other to turn him. I had a shot of pethidine, and one stitch. That was the sum total of the interference. They [midwife and doctor] were stalwart. They enormously respected my wishes. I felt I'd escaped by the skin of my teeth. With him being the wrong way round, and me in full labour, they'd probably have done a Caesarian. I had a great birth – by chance.

Others were pleased with what they saw as the relative ease of their labour. A sixth of the group thought theirs good enough to remark on. Some women saw their birth as having transformed their lives. Birth as therapy, birth as change, birth as growth: there was almost no end to the meanings given by women to their experiences. Sue had a second degree tear, which gave her trouble for a year. But this did not alter her perception of the birth:

Afterwards I felt that she [the midwife] had helped me through a very profound experience, perhaps the most profound experience of my life . . . It was a very sacred event. There was a feeling of new life.

It was her first baby. Nora says she walked the earth in total harmony for a year afterwards: 'It was such a profound, essential experience that I felt it connected me to the whole world.'

For women who had been traumatized by a previous hospital experience, their home birth was healing. It helped them to integrate painful and humiliating memories, they believed, easing their sense of violation, failure and bruised self-esteem. Brenda describes how therapeutic it was for her to expiate the trauma of earlier births:

There was no unfinished business after Paul's birth, unlike the hospital ones. When it was over, it was over. I look back on it as a very positive and happy experience, with healing qualities.

Deborah had been given electric shock treatment for severe postnatal depression after the birth of her second child in hospital (see Chapter 2). She is explicit about how this, the birth of her third child, restored her to herself:

> I was pleased I'd gone and done it. I'd almost have liked to have gone back to St Mary's, and done it right. All the yearning and aggravation that I'd had after Stephen's birth went.

Some women reported a sense of enhanced self-esteem. They felt the birth had added something to their lives, to their sense of themselves. It was an unexpected bonus that cut across differences in women's social circumstances. Whether they were married, middle-class and unemployed, like Tríona ('the birth was a builder of confidence for me in my life'), or separated and running a one-parent household on welfare, like Nuala, the effect was the same. She says the birth was the best thing that ever happened to her:

> It changed the way I thought about myself ... I had a sense of well-being affirmed by the birth, a more positive sense of myself, because I had mastered it.

For many women, the days and weeks after birth could be difficult. It was a trying time, not made any easier by the lack of household help, by the non-appearance of health visitors. It was all too easy for women to give up on breast-feeding. Or to become depressed. The more serious the depression, the less help women got, or so it seemed. Feelings of isolation and alienation were common at this time. Many women felt bereft of support from the health services. It was almost as though, having broken the rules, you could expect nothing.

Were they risking their lives, and those of their babies, as they had been told? There were no deaths. Just four per cent of mothers had to go to hospital for complications. And three per cent of babies were admitted for jaundice or anaemia, including one seen as an out-patient. No baby had a seizure, a sign of 'cerebral irritation', during the first 48 hours. No baby was brain-damaged. No mother reported long-term developmental problems with her child. Neither was the group entirely what doctors would describe as 'low-risk'.[27] Small babies were more common than might have been expected. So were congenital disorders. As many as six per cent of babies were small, and four per cent were born with congenital problems. By definition, no births ended up in hospital, as the listing from which the sample was taken did not include hospital transfers. This is a serious limitation on the findings. However, there is nothing in these results to justify the attitude of health professionals who intimidated some of these women during their pregnancies, asking them if they wanted to kill their babies.

Most women were very satisfied with the way things went. They felt they got the kind of birth they wanted, that they were looked after by midwives and doctors who knew them, that their care was personal. They talked about how natural the birth was at home, how it made a difference not having to go through the standard hospital procedures, like being examined every two hours. They talked about their sense of being in control at home, and of feeling free and physically unconfined.

Many of the women talked about their husbands' role in the birth and about how much it meant to both of them. They described the warmth and closeness that resulted from their other children being able to come in straightaway to see the baby, and everyone sitting up together in bed. They stressed the gentleness of the birth for the baby, and spoke about the happiness of being able to hold their babies for hours afterwards, without interruption. These were their priorities in birth.

We buried the placenta in the garden, and planted a tree on it. We brought the tree with us when we moved house [Bridget].

Acts of Defiance

To many people, having a baby on your own without a midwife or a doctor to look after you sounds crazy, risky, way out-of-line. A number of women within the group decided to go ahead without professional help. Faced with either going to hospital or staying at home on their own with their partners, 11 per cent of women – their backs up against the wall – made such a decision.

How many women choose to go it alone in countries with a hospital-based system of maternity care? The answer is that we do not know: the research has yet to be done. Most of these births took place in the South-west. The two maternity units servicing the region have since closed. So had they wished to, neither Jane, Lise, Jenny nor Judy, all of whom had a short labour, would have made it to hospital today.

None of them had lay midwives. There are now no lay midwives in Ireland. After the introduction of the Midwives' Bill in 1931, the handywomen, who were part and parcel of life in most communities, gradually stopped practising.[1] And lay midwifery as a by-product of what has been called the 'birth culture' never developed in Ireland, as it did in North America.[2]

In the eyes of the state, to have a non-attended birth by choice is grossly irresponsible. In England, delivering your own baby has been criminalized.[3] Looked at from women's point of view, unattended birth highlights the gap between supply and demand, between the kind of maternity service offered by the state, and what women – some women – want.

What made them do it? Sometimes it can be difficult to disen-tangle personal motives from the doublespeak of the state. Women do what they do against a background of sustained opposition from the health care system to home birth. Community midwifery is legal, but there are only a handful of midwives working outside the hospitals. The Voluntary Health Insurance Board, a body with a virtual monopoly on private health care insurance, refused to recognize midwives as inde-pendent practitioners. Women are legally entitled to a mater-nity service at home, but the state pays midwives a pittance. Women have to pay the difference between the state fee and the private fees being charged by independent midwives. Some women just do not have the money.

Nearly everyone in this group of 15 is alienated from the health care system. There was some ambivalence about midwives. Some women had their personal reasons for doing what they did. And some women talked more freely than others.

To Gwen, unattended birth offered the prospect of complete control over an event that she regards as spiritual. For other women, it was an opportunity to rebuild a rocky relationship. Honor and her partner undertook it as a joint project, as marriage therapy.

Other women seem to have been driven to it, as though the decision to go it alone was almost taken under duress. Simone feels so alienated from the state and its institutions that to expect her to give birth in one would be unrealistic. Felicity has been badly hurt by the hospital system. Gillian has no faith left in it, either.

Then there are the women for whom having an unattended birth is simply how it was on the night. Circumstances inter-lock, such as short labour, the absence of a local midwife, a reluctance to go to hospital, transport difficulties, and, last but not least, money problems. Jenny was let down by her doctor at the eleventh hour. Pamela left it until the last minute to make up her mind, and then found there was no time to go to hospital.

Finally, unattended birth can have a fundamental appeal. For some women, if not for all, there may be the lure of the primitive, the ultimate birth experience. More readily acknowledged by women is the V-sign to the medical establishment, the supreme revolt against obstetrics.

⤳

Parents

Most of the women, and men, in this small group are from outside Ireland. Many of them are English. They have been living in Ireland for a number of years. What brought them to the country? Some were attracted by what they saw as a Celtic culture going back to the dawn of pre-history, endowed with a fabulous mythological past. Felicity, for example, is interested in the old earth religions. Others were impressed by the seemingly casual, easy-going nature of life in Ireland, where, they felt, the state does not breathe down your neck. Simone and Jacques, from France, were particularly struck by the fact that in Ireland they do not have to carry identity papers. What they may not know is that, to the native mind, every blade of grass that grows in rural Ireland has been counted.

Almost everyone in this group lives deep in the heart of the country. 'Why do you think we live here?' Jane asks. 'Draw our own water? It's nature, the natural life.' Ireland never had an industrial revolution, and the density of population is low by European standards. The landscape of the island is reminiscent of a Constable painting – lush, romantic, pastoral. To industrial refugees, the prospect of being able to live in a green world is magical. But the green world can be desolate, barren, remote. Neighbours can be few and far between. Roads can be narrow, twisting boreens with grass growing up through the tarmac, if there is any.

For the past 10 years, Simone and Jacques have been living in a mobile home without facilities, half a field from the nearest unmarked boreen. It is the hidden Ireland, just a few miles from the coast, the Ireland tourists never see. Together with another couple, they formed their own tiny enclave ten years ago. They survive, not on state benefits, but by making baskets which they sell during the summer months to tourists.

Living in a remote homestead, far from the centres of maternity care, can have certain consequences. Lise, from Holland, explains: 'We were living a 10 minute walk off the road. There is no way I could walk down that track in labour.' Although only a few miles from a village, Cindy and her husband also lived in an isolated area. Like others, they had no transport of any kind. No transport and no phone.

Living in makeshift or temporary accommodation such as a mobile home, or in a formerly abandoned cottage without facilities such as running water or electricity, is par for the course. Lise and Rudolf were living in a tent. Another Dutch couple, in the throes of building their own house, were living in what amounted to a garden shed, unwired and unplumbed.

Lise and Rudolf are the only ones who tried to live without money, to be self-sufficient. It is impossible, Lise says. Material hardship is part of life for these people. Some are on the dole. For others, not being on welfare is a matter of principle. Everyone was entitled to free medical – and maternity – care on income grounds.

Felicity, who is from the south of England, is the only one in the group with a nomadic life-style. She and her family live in a horse-drawn wagon, just like the ones Irish travellers used to have, wintering in an encampment in a field near the ruins of an ancient abbey, and spending the summer on the outskirts of a southern port city.

These families stand out like a sore thumb among their conservative, Catholic neighbours, and contact is minimal. 'Standing out' in rural Ireland, where the same families have been living on the same farms for generations, is not difficult. With the exception of Siobhán, a native of the village where she lived and Una, who had moved from Belfast to the West, the hippie label is something these women, and their families, probably have to live with, to varying degrees.

❧

Falling on Deaf Ears

Studies show that in the absence of a home birth service, some parents go ahead without professional assistance.[4] In parts of North America, home birth has been driven underground.[5] Senior public health doctors in Ireland are acutely aware of the 'problem' of unattended births. The problem has no solution, as they see it. You cannot make someone go to hospital. Their feeling is one of extreme anxiety lest something go wrong, an anxiety that stems in part from fear of litigation.

Women in this small group were only too well aware of the attitude of the local health board, and most did not even apply for a service. Judy is one of two women who tried, and failed, to get what she was entitled to from the state. Her second child was born at home, with a midwife, in England. She was having her second unattended birth – her fourth child – in Ireland:

> I went to a lot of trouble sussing out a midwife. I wrote to the health board. They say in their booklet that they provide a home birth service. But they said that there was no service, that there were no midwives.

Her letter only resulted in a visit from a public health nurse, who advised her to have her baby in hospital. This advice did nothing to alter Judy's views:

> Maybe it was reckless of me, but I felt I ought to be able to have that baby at home. We wanted to have the baby at home so much that it overrode our fears.

To these women, the machinery of the state is off-putting. Forms are all-powerful, and their power is negative:

> The health board make it very complicated. The midwife lives in one county and we live in another. You needed to

go to them three months before the birth, [to apply] so they could have their forms [Pamela].

Out of date information could also be a factor. Fíona, who is Irish, planned to have her first baby at home and got a list of midwives from her local community health centre. However, the only one who was practising was herself having a baby. Fíona's local doctor said he would perform the delivery, but in labour she was tricked, she says, into going to hospital by a locum who told her she might haemorrhage. In hospital, she believes she was duped again:

> The nurse said 'I'm going to give you something that's good for you.' I thought it was glucose, but it wasn't. It was to speed up the labour. I couldn't control the breathing with the pain.

Although opposed to the idea of taking pethidine in labour, she eventually took it.

Honor, too, had a bad birth, in an English hospital: 'I'd had a slight tear which they'd stitched. The stitching was very humiliating. And afterwards, it was very uncomfortable.' Her sense of indignity is echoed by Cindy, an American with bitter memories of her first birth in an Irish hospital:

> The staff were very abrupt. I was left there. They didn't tell me anything. Just came along and poked a finger up. With the memory of that, there was no way I was going into hospital when I found I was pregnant.

Unlike most of the others in the group, Jane is reluctant to speak. She and her partner clashed with local health officers: 'We were *persona non grata* with the health board. No doctor would take us.' They were wounded by the system, casualties in the on-going war between the health board and women who wanted a home birth. In the medical literature, people are sometimes graded according to their willingness to take doctors' advice. Patients who are slow to do as they are told are considered to be 'poorly compliant'. Jane and Tim were undoubtedly regarded as 'poor compliers'.

Such labelling goes right to the heart of the matter. To the providers of the service, it is those on the receiving end – women – who are the problem. The difficulty, as health professionals see it, is that women – some women – are refusing to have their babies in hospital. The problem, as far as women are concerned, is with the service. They feel that doctors have taken over from women. Gillian, who is Irish, sums it up: 'They extract the baby from you. The worst thing about hospital is not that they do it to you, it is that you allow them to do it to you. You relinquish yourself to them.' Asked what made them go ahead on their own, ten women say that it was because they could not get a midwife or a doctor at home. As women see it, the problem is that they have to admit themselves to the potentially dangerous environment of a hospital in order to get the services of a midwife or a doctor.[6]

Felicity had always gone to hospital for the protection of the child, she says, 'but after the twins died . . .' The twins' birth was her fifth; she does not elaborate very much on their delivery. All she will say is that it was 'so cold. I had to be cut. They damaged a nerve. It was awful.' Physical scars fade. About their deaths, at two and four months respectively, she says nothing. She had her next child, unattended, in a Welsh valley, having tried and failed to get a midwife. She does not feel she can talk to doctors:

> They just look up their MIMS [a drugs directory]. It's their insensitivity that puts me off. Like they are automated, forgetting to be human.

It is difficult not to see unattended births as part and parcel of a revolt by women against modern medicine. All illness is a cry for help, Felicity believes. A cry for attention. The failure of the system encompasses more than maternity care. Gwen, for instance, believes that doctors, generally, only tell people enough to get them to do as they are told: 'They don't allow you to take responsibility. They just want to take over and do it their way.' Like many women who are not well off, Una is deeply alienated from an obstetrical system that demands only obedience, as far as she can see: 'Doctors are usually men. They take over women's bodies.' In what Ann Oakley has called 'the user-provider debate' on the maternity services,[7] the class war could be difficult to distinguish from the gender gap. 'Doctors keep people in ignorance to control them,' she says, angrily.

ぺ

Mixed Feelings

We asked informally, but there were just no midwives. If there'd been a midwife, we would have had one. I suppose I liked the idea of just Keith and myself. We felt quite strong about it.

Necessity can be stretched, sometimes, to fit other needs. Honor is frank about the fact that she and Keith were having serious emotional and financial difficulties. Planning this birth together offered a chance to improve things between them. 'I'd had two good births and two good pregnancies [medically], otherwise I'd never have done it,' she says. 'We felt that it was morally right,' Keith adds. 'We were taking full responsibility for the birth.' He is the only one within the group to bring up the ethics of having an unattended birth by choice.

Unattended birth can be part necessity, part choice, part lifestyle. 'You've got to understand the way we were living,' Cindy says. She is the only one to underline just how much home birth was a part of their lifestyle:

It was so remote. Home birth was almost the norm. No one had really had any problems, so we were getting these positive feedbacks. It was really, like, us against the world.

Things look very different from the edge. The decision becomes whether or not to come back in to the centre, to drive (or walk) down that twisting boreen, deeply cratered and overgrown with grass, miles off the main road, hours from a maternity hospital . . .

Honor and Cindy belonged to the same tiny community of people who had come from elsewhere to live in this remote part of Ireland, on the edge of fields of stone where crops of wild flowers grow in the summer. Like Honor ('a big influence'), Cindy saw the birth as a way of improving a troubled marriage: 'It really did bring us closer together, planning, arranging everything. So we didn't really want anybody else.' She later resented her husband's role in the birth:

It was really his trip. He was incredibly arrogant about it. As far as he was concerned, it was no problem.

She makes it sound like there was an element of machismo in the way he acted. He was one of the few men – apart from Honor's husband – who delivered his own child and this gave him 'a political pivoting point' in the community: 'Everyone else had had a midwife or a woman who had delivered babies.' Motives are almost always mixed: 'And it was also, like, it was part of growing up for me, 'cos I had lived a very sheltered life, very protected.' Finally, there is always the background against which people make their decisions: 'There were no midwives, anyway.'

If home birth is part of what has been called the 'counterculture', there is one country in Europe where it is not counter to the mainstream. Having a home birth in Holland, where a third of all babies are born at home, is quite normal, Lise says, speaking of her native country. For Lise, having her third child and living miles from nowhere, there was another factor: 'I give birth so quickly,' she says, 'there is no time to go to hospital.'

Doctors frequently put forward the view that, in choosing to give birth at home, women are being selfish, that they care more about themselves than they do about their babies. But it is precisely because women care about their babies that they choose home birth. The baby's first impressions are important, Ingrid, who is also from the Netherlands, believes. 'He is coming from warm red surroundings'. She talks about the trauma of birth, insisting that 'It does not have to be like that. You can have a happy baby.' Like Cindy, she believes that birth affects us for the rest of our lives.

Ingrid would have preferred to have a midwife: 'We had no choice except to do it ourselves or go into hospital.' She had her first baby in Ireland, unattended. 'The first time it was different. I did not know what it was like. But when you know what can go wrong . . .' This time it was a forced choice: 'It is better to have a midwife.' She is not the only woman in this small group who changed her mind about unattended birth.

Where you decide to have your baby can depend to some extent on how you see the world. For Simone and Jacques 'the intimacy and the spirituality of birth are taken away in hospital.' They both believe that birth is the entry of the spirit made flesh into the world. They cannot bring themselves to desecrate it by subjecting it to hospital. They believe in predestination, in the teachings of the German philosopher, Rudolf Steiner. 'Everyone is destined according to his place of birth,' Jacques explains. One of their children was born in a remote, mountainous region. Another was born by the sea: 'They have developed accordingly,' Simone maintains.

Birth becomes very important to some men. To men who take on the responsibility of acting as midwife to their partners in labour, birth generally matters more rather than less. Jacques has a strong sense of fatherhood. According to him, parenthood is damaged in hospital: 'The state kills the spiritual bond between mother and child, and father and child.' To call them a united couple would be an understatement. Jacques speaks for Simone, and Simone speaks for Jacques, though not as often.

Like Fíona, Simone feels she has been betrayed by health professionals in the past. The public health nurse said she would deliver her first baby, then called a doctor instead at the last minute. Women need help in childbirth. Silent support, preferably at a distance, might be the answer, as they see it: 'The ideal, maybe, would be to have the midwife at a discreet distance, in the background, so that she would be there if needed.' Simone echoes Keith's words. They are attempting to reconcile the idea of professional support with the notion of personal autonomy.

Gwen also believes that birth is too important to allow it to take place in hospital:

> Birth is spiritual. Starlight was born in a tepee. We had built it ourselves. Some people might think that was weird, but to us, it was a kind of temple.

Birth is sacred. There is no sense here, as there is with other women, of having been driven to it by a harsh, uncaring system, devoid of warmth and humanity. For Gwen, it was a positive choice. She is ambivalent about midwives, however:

> I chose to have Terry deliver her. Maybe if there was a midwife of like mind, who would give us support in a professional way, it would be easier for Terry than having all the responsibility for it.

To couples who go down this particular road, being able to do it together, without the limitations they ascribe to professionals, is important. The desire for a midwife who would not dominate, who would stay in the background, comes up again and again.

Sometimes our motives for doing things may not be clear to ourselves. 'If anything went wrong,' Fiona explains, 'I knew I could get to a hospital ... You should have a trained midwife.' But the feeling that you need someone professional can co-exist with other feelings. Asked if she would have an unattended birth again, she replies, 'Yes, if I was in good health, if there were no problems.' The safest thing, Fiona feels, is to have professional help. So why risk an unattended birth? The reason she gives for not taking painkillers in labour may have something to do with it: 'You're testing yourself as a human being. To see what the limits are.'

Seeing what the limits are may be one of the attractions –
acknowledged or otherwise – of unattended birth.

ↄ

Hit and Miss

Feelings can be acknowledged or unacknowledged, resolved
or unresolved. Sometimes the decision not to go to hospital
was touch and go. Within the group of 15 unattended births,
several owed as much to contingency or chance as they did to
intention or resolve.

The border between an unplanned fast labour at home and
an intentional unattended home birth can be a narrow one.
Pamela both wanted and did not want a home birth. She both
wanted and did not want a hospital birth:

> I was going to wait and see how I felt when the time came.
> I suppose I really wanted a home delivery, but up to a week
> or two before the birth, I still didn't know whether I'd go
> to hospital or stay at home. The doctor didn't really want
> me to stay at home, but he was prepared to come if I
> needed him. I had booked into the hospital.

Within the entire group, Pamela's is the only home birth you
could call 'accidental on purpose':

> It was around twelve at night, and I thought, maybe. By
> about one, I said, definitely. My husband got back around
> twelve thirty. I started timing the contractions. I didn't
> want to go to hospital if they were only ten minutes apart.
> You could be in there for hours!
>
> At about one thirty I told Ian to phone the doctor. The
> contractions were coming every three minutes. The
> doctor said 'Can't you get her into hospital?' Ian was still
> on the phone, and I was shouting down at him, telling him
> he'd miss it if he didn't get off the phone! Ian ran upstairs

and saw the head about to come out. He stopped it so I wouldn't tear.

The birth was a joint effort: 'My husband was working for a doctor at the time. He knew about these things.' To go or not to go, that is the decision. Pamela postponed hers until it was too late. Had there been a midwife, she adds, she would definitely have booked one.

Jenny, a second generation alternative born in Ireland of English parents, was also in two minds about staying at home: 'I knew as soon as I went into labour that it felt right.' The public health nurse told her home birth was not on the service, that there were not any midwives to do it. Her doctor told her he would do the delivery, and she persuaded her mother to act as her midwife. Calling the doctor meant deciding to stay at home. But when it happened, he was not on duty, and his partner refused to come out. Faced with the choice of going to hospital or having an unattended birth at home, she opted for the latter.

The stakes were high. She had lost her first baby when she was three months old in a fire in a mobile home. When Jenny was five weeks pregnant, she had her appendix taken out: 'They said I'd probably lose the baby.' She was 21.

∽

Antenatal Care

Regular antenatal care was not the norm. Honor made extensive preparations for the birth, but they did not include antenatal care: 'I knew if I went to a doctor, he would have sent me into hospital,' she explains. To these people, it seems as though the medical system has been reduced to a form of social control. Ann Oakley makes the point, however, that controlling women has always been an intrinsic part of antenatal care.[8] Simone had no antenatal care, either. A visit to a doctor early in pregnancy did little for her confidence in the medical profession: 'We went to a doctor to find out if I was pregnant, and he told me I had a kidney problem. That was the only time.'

Half of the group did not see a midwife or a doctor until they were seven months pregnant, or more. Women who do without regular antenatal care usually make one visit to a doctor or a midwife, at the end of pregnancy. The purpose of this visit is to rule out the possibility that the baby is breech, or in some other position that would make the birth difficult or even impossible. Fortunately, the vast majority of babies are perfectly positioned to make their entry into the world. A transverse lie is rare. Gwen saw a doctor twice in the last two weeks. She explains why she did not go earlier: 'I was put off doctors in England.' Had she known what this doctor was like, she implies, she would have seen him earlier: 'He is quite unusual. He told us the baby was in the right position, that she was the right size.'

Not everyone left it until near the end. Ingrid went to a local doctor for her antenatal care from five months. Jane got her antenatal care from a midwife whom she knew. Fíona is one of two women who went to a public hospital clinic for her antenatal care. They made her feel guilty, she says:

They asked me, 'What are you going to do if the baby's breech? If the baby's blue? If the cord is around the neck?'

2)

In Training

Every day, from the fourth month onwards, Judy took raspberry leaf tea and caulophyllum, a homeopathic, to tone the womb and to make labour easier. Raspberry leaf tea is a favourite. Pamela took squaw's root as well: 'It makes you looser and the contractions lighter.' Honor combined raspberry leaf tea with calcium. Taking calcium, some believe, lightens contractions and makes them more 'efficient'.

Like nearly everyone else in this group, Lise seemed to be in very good health at the time of her pregnancy:

I was physically very strong. I'd been drinking blackberry tea all during my pregnancy. I only found out later that this strengthens the muscles of the womb.

Minding your diet, taking supplements such as calcium or berry teas, is one kind of preparation. Physically toning the body in preparation for what many women assume will be a marathon, is another: 'If you can run up the mountain, then you can give birth,' Lise maintains. But for women with young children and few, if any, of the basic facilities, birth exercises were not an option. Asked about exercises for pregnancy and birth, Honor says: 'I had four children to look after, aged six, five, four and three, so that was enough for me!' Their caravan had electricity, but no water.

Cindy is the only one who did pain threshold exercises: 'Like where he'd grip my wrist very, very tightly, and I would breathe through it.' Doing something that reinforces the expectation of pain in labour may not be such a good idea. Cindy had a difficult labour.

༂

Preparing to Go it Alone

Most women did not have a second pair of hands to look after them during labour – someone to hold their hand, to encourage them, and to deliver the baby. In other countries, in unattended births, studies show that the baby's father is usually registered as the main attendant; this may be a device to protect the lay midwife involved.[9] Only 4 out of the 15 women in this group had access to another woman at this essentially female time.

How can a couple prepare themselves for delivering a baby? Judy answers succinctly:

We knew how to get the baby to breathe, if she wasn't breathing. And I knew about a retained placenta. I sterilized everything. What else was there we could do?

Farming experience is mentioned. Calves and goats can have cord problems, too: 'It's the same with calves, isn't it?' Pamela asks. Her husband is one of two men in this group with a background in farming.

Experience in human midwifery as opposed to animal husbandry is more difficult to come by. Men's experience of midwifery was usually confined to the birth of their own children – seven couples had done it before. There was little suggestion that the women helpers were more experienced.

Asked how her partner prepared for the birth, Lise replies, 'He read all the books.' Reading was often all men could do by way of preparation. Honor explains how they had a very good knowledge:

Keith even knew how to check the cord before the baby came out, to make sure it wasn't around the neck. We'd got everything on the list from *Spiritual Midwifery*. Keith [a mechanic] had even made a homemade mucus-sucker! I'd got sterile sheets and we had this feather bed all ready. We'd even boiled five gallons of water – we were wondering what to do with it afterwards!

Preparations for the birth could be complicated. Cindy talks about how difficult it was, in a stressed marriage, to work out in advance how things should be done when the time came: 'Things weren't very easy between us. Nobody wanted to push the other.'

'We got a friend who lived in a house on standby with a car,' Gwen says. Gwen was not the only one having an unattended birth, living in the back of beyond without transport. Of the 15 women in the group, 8 were in this position. Some did not even have friends in houses on standby with cars.

Supplies and equipment could pose their own problems. Fíona went to a Dublin health care supplier's to buy a home

birth kit; they didn't want to sell one to her. 'It was really difficult to get cord clamps,' Ingrid recalls, 'just one set instead of a
thousand! And surgical gloves.'

For Simone and Jacques, preparation for the birth centred
around spiritual reading. 'Birth is a manifestation of the divine
will,' Jacques says. Books on childbirth, according to Simone,
are based on fear. They concentrate on the 'mechanics' of
labour, and she wanted no 'gymnastics'. Their stance, ultimately, is one of personal powerlessness in the face of God.
Childbirth, Jacques says, is a matter of life and death, both for
the baby and for the mother. How did he learn midwifery? He
tried to read some of the books, he says, but they were
confusing:

> You could not possibly take it all in, the different posi-
> tions, and so on. It is not in the head that you learn it, but
> in the solar plexus. It is intuitive.

He is the only one who raises the question as to how far
midwifery can be learned from books.

ॐ

Psyching Up

Antenatal visits are expected to provide the comfort of
knowing that all is well during the months of pregnancy.
Without them, you may have to look to within yourself for
reassurance. How did Honor, who did not see a doctor or a
midwife, feel in those last weeks about the possibility of something going wrong? 'I had premonitions and dreams,' she
replies, unhesitatingly. 'I saw him safe and sound in a dream,
so I knew he was going to be okay.' Her feelings of confidence
and security were not entirely unmixed, however: 'I suppose I
was slightly apprehensive,' she admits. Within the larger
group, as well as worrying about the possibility of something
going wrong, women often worried about pain. But Honor

did not. She knew a woman in Wales who had given birth to six children on her own, without anyone: 'I felt as though I could run off into the woods and have it by myself.'

Within this group, there was a belief in dreams, an emphasis on intuition, a reliance on supra-rational knowledge. Simone heard voices: 'I got clear messages telling me the baby was in the right position.' Most women do not have that kind of faith. For them, birth is a time when you stand alone. Ingrid remarks that in India women squat behind the bushes to give birth; she identifies the psychology of fear surrounding birth in the West:

> Women are afraid. The books and the articles make them afraid. Home births are usual in Holland. You go to hospital if you are ill.

Ingrid believes that if you think about trouble, you attract it. It is easier for women to give birth at home, she feels,[10] because in hospital, fear of birth is pathogenic. It causes complications. Asked how she felt about the prospect of going it alone, Lise replies: 'We just had no choice in the matter.' She continues: 'If the baby wasn't in the right position, I would have gone to hospital. That's the only thing you can tell in advance.' Ingrid and Lise were both pregnant at the same time; the nearest hospital was 45 minutes' drive away. They used to psyche each other up: 'We used to talk about it,' Ingrid recalls, 'convince each other that everything was going to be all right.'

Asked how she felt about the birth coming to the end of pregnancy, Pamela's response is matter-of-fact: 'I was confident. The hospital wasn't that far, and the doctor was there as a back-up.' The possibility of the cord being knotted, or tightly wrapped around the baby's neck, is something some women worry about: 'The cord was probably the only thing. My husband was prepared for this.' If your husband is to be your midwife, having faith in him is essential. Gwen says she felt confident:

> About a week before the birth, I had a day of feeling nervous, of feeling that I couldn't do it . . . I had total faith

in Terry. He knew it all by heart. He had really researched it all.

Cindy was not frightened, either:

> I was incredibly healthy during the pregnancy. I went to the regular clinics in the hospital. The baby was in a good position . . . I really got into that headspace, reading those testimonials in *Spiritual Midwifery*.[11] And he read the technical bit. I trusted him.

It is clear from what Cindy says that, while reading gave her confidence, it was her reliance on her husband, her faith in his ability to tackle technically demanding projects, that counted. However, she raises the difficulty of seeking help in the event of an emergency, in the absence of a phone, without a car and without another adult to call on: 'The only thing was we'd no car. We were just hoping nothing would go wrong.' There was something else. Early in pregnancy she had had keyhole surgery to remove scar tissue from an old womb operation, before she knew she was pregnant. Obstetricians would have considered that there was some risk that her womb might rupture.

Judy was relying on herself. She talks about personal limits, about where to draw the line:

> If something had gone wrong, I would have gone to hospital. If the labour was premature, if it hadn't followed the pattern of my previous labours, or if I was anxious or frightened, I would have gone to hospital.

She was a 'bit anxious' before the birth, she says. 'I only realized afterwards how anxious I'd been.' The doctor, she says, was 'very positive, very encouraging'. If doctors have the power to reduce women's confidence, they also have the ability to increase it.

Some women were told by their doctors that they would come in an emergency. Gwen says her doctor was in a very difficult position: 'He said he would come out if anything went wrong, but he didn't want to take responsibility for the birth.' Gillian's doctor said he would come to check the afterbirth, too. General practitioners can find themselves caught between the demands of their patients on the one hand, and the wrath of their medical colleagues on the other. Lise says her doctor encouraged her to go ahead with the birth: he was subsequently threatened with the withdrawal of his licence, her partner observed.[12]

Do unattended births ever end in tragedy? Fíona relates a story she had previously heard:

> I knew of a couple of home births in the country, both unattended. On one of them, the cord was around the baby's neck, and the baby died. Things might have turned out differently if they'd had a midwife.

⅔

Birth and Beyond

The night before I felt very different – emotionally – although there were no physical signs. I woke up at five o'clock in the morning, in labour. We got up and did the usual things, like lighting the stove. I was getting a contraction every forty minutes. I couldn't lie down. I had to keep moving. So we went for a walk, up to the top of the mountain, and watched the dawn! It was great. Then we got Sunshine [their two-year-old] her breakfast.

It got more painful, for a few contractions. I didn't know how long it was going to go on for. Terry called our friend. After that it got very intense. The contractions were coming more quickly and it wasn't really painful. I used the breathing I'd learnt in rebirthing, connected breathing. Moving around, even swinging my foot or my arm, that really helped.

In transition I had a change of energy. I was really in control. The birth was easy. I felt really powerful. I could really feel all that birthing energy come out. Sunshine said 'Oh look, there's a baby coming out of Gwen's bum!' and carried on eating her breakfast! She just slid out all together, in one piece, with the waters. They broke as she came out.

She was lovely when she was born, covered in that stuff that's on their skin. It was really thick. I could see it. It was like her skin was soaking it in, absorbing the nourishment. I could see her skin changing colour. She was quite pink when she was born. She cried briefly. She was fine. She was lying on me. That was the best part of it, in a way, being with her.

The cord had all these rainbow colours around it. We didn't cut it until it looked like it had shrivelled up and stopped pulsating. The placenta took about two hours. Hilda and Terry wanted me to get up but I wanted to lie down. Eventually, I got up and it came away, just like that. I used shepherd's purse, a homeopathic thing, to help it come away. It helps the blood – what do you call them – [platelets] not to stick together into little lumps . . . I really enjoyed the birth.

Gwen had a four-hour labour, which is about average within the larger group.

Cindy's labour was more difficult. She pinpoints the moment when everything went to pieces, the point where she stopped believing in her ability to give birth:

I wasn't dilating as quickly as I should have been. By mid-afternoon, I was only two or three fingers [dilated]. So I got really down. It was, like, he didn't know what to do. So he said, 'Okay, so we've failed, right? If you want me to take you to hospital, I will.' And I was, like, 'Take me away out of here.' I wanted my mother, anything, just not to be here. The breathing got a big ragged. I lost it. We just got to a point where we were no longer able to sustain each other. We were exhausted. We couldn't carry on. I needed someone very strong, and he wasn't able to be that.

The arrival of a female friend changed everything:

> A friend of mine came in. She took one look at me, and got me up out of the chair. I said, 'I can't walk.' They walked me backwards and forwards in the kitchen. Up and down. Then, suddenly, I said, 'Stop, I think the head is coming down.' Rory was fine. He was serene, calm, very present.

Cindy, who is American, needed that second person to be there. In difficult births, there is often this crisis of confidence, when a woman can feel she is just not going to be able to do it. Gillian, who is Irish, also doubted her own ability: 'I thought she would never come out.' Giving birth is not necessarily instinctive. In the sense of innate knowledge, women have lost it: 'They had to tell me how to breathe,' Gillian says. 'They had to show me how to push. I was pushing up instead of down.'

Each labour is different. How you give birth depends on who you are, on how you see birth, on how you see life. The early part of Simone's labour was calm and visionary: 'I was conscious of powers, of beings all around me. I could feel the angels all around me. I had this vision of a stork.' Her labour got more and more difficult:

> I could feel the baby wasn't coming down. It [her labour] was very strong. Jacques helped me. At a certain point, I lost confidence. I wanted to go to hospital. I had to walk down the track. It was a stormy night. I was bent over, with Jacques supporting me. I fell in the mud three times before we reached the car. He couldn't start the car. Then I called, 'Jacques, it's coming!' I was in the back seat and the car had only two doors. He came out easily in a few pushes.

By then, Simone was exhausted: she had had a 16-hour labour. Her mother had just arrived from France; she had not known her daughter was pregnant, and she did not approve of home births. But Simone can identify the precise point at which things began to go wrong: 'I suffered so much that I decided I'd had enough.' She blames herself. For her, willing something to happen is setting oneself against the will of God.

Una, the second Irishwoman in this group of 15, also had a hard labour. They did not know why he was not coming out, she says:

> It was very painful. I thought I'd never get him out. If I'd been in hospital, I'd have had a Caesarian section! He had a big head. Larry had to turn him, first one shoulder, and then the other. There was a lot of pushing.

At 5 ft 2 in, she was having a 10½ lb baby.

Labour can be demanding without being a nightmare. 'Mergey and fairly violent' is how Felicity describes hers, towards the end. She relates how she gave birth virtually on her own, without any tangible support from her partner (who is nine years younger than she is). Asked how painful it was, she replies:

> Fairly excruciating. It was strong from the beginning. It started in the evening after dinner. He was born at dawn, by the fire. We'd brought out blankets and cushions, earlier – I wanted to go outside. He played the guitar. We made tea. I smoked fags. Afterwards, it was really quiet. We all just crashed out.

She gave birth in a field.

In Ireland, being born in the caul, or amniotic sac, is believed to be a sign of good luck. In an unattended birth, a caul, although not classified by doctors as a complication, could amount to one. Jane's baby was born with the membranes covering her face. Her partner explains how you deal with them, by drawing them down over the baby's face, pinching her nostrils at the same time, to prevent fluid getting into her airways.

In labour, the only language you want to speak is your first one. Irish is Siobhán's first language: in hospital for the birth of her child, she discovered that no one spoke Irish. If it had not been for that, she says, she would have gone back. She went into labour at the antenatal clinic in the hospital, said nothing to anyone, got the bus, walked the three miles to her house, made a cup of tea, and gave birth an hour later. It was a two-hour journey on a bad road. Siobhán points out how she could have had the baby on the bus: her labours are short. The idea that a midwife or a doctor might come to her house to look after her in labour has never occurred to Siobhán. Her next-door neighbour, who has ten children herself, came in to look after her, as she always did. She was having her fifth child. Her birth is a throwback to the time when handywomen delivered babies. Siobhán smiles at the idea that her husband might have had anything to do with the birth. He would come in to their bedroom only after he heard the baby crying, she says. Her eighty-year-old mother-in-law was there, too: she had nine children at home. The lastborn was referred to in Irish as *croitheadh mála* ('the remnants of the bag'). Their world is a harsh one.

Jenny's birth was 'very easy, very smooth'. She makes it sound effortless:

They were like little rushes first. Like a tickling in my tummy. It got stronger in the bath, then suddenly it got very intense. It was like he was pushing himself out. I am not sure if pain is the right word. It wasn't what I'd have thought of as pain.

Lise, who is Dutch, had what doctors would call a 'precipitate' labour:

For the last six weeks, I had been having very strong contractions. The night before, I couldn't sleep all night, although I was very relaxed. I got up early to make some porridge. I put the kettle on to boil. Then I got this enormous contraction, and I went 'Ah!', like that. I went upstairs. The water bag was coming out. Rudolf almost had to put his hand in the boiling water, to sterilize the scissors to puncture it. By the time the water was boiled, she was born.

Her labour lasted 10 minutes: 'Everything happened so quickly, there was no time to do anything. It was chaotic.'

Honor felt that she was 'in total control' of her labour:

I just said to myself, 'I'm going for it'. Keith was checking my dilatation ['I was directing the movie' – Keith]. I didn't really feel as if I was there at all. I used to imagine that I was riding these waves, with the contractions! I kept on telling myself there is an end to this. At one point Keith told me not to push, because I wasn't fully dilated.

I pushed him out. It was the first time I'd seen a baby come out. There were bubbles coming out of his mouth as he came out. The head came first, then a couple of pushes later, plop! The rest came. He was making these arm movements, as if he was still inside. He seemed a bit panicky. He just lay there on my belly. He didn't cry for a couple of days.

꒜

Calling a Doctor

Jenny's afterbirth took nearly an hour and a half, and they called the doctor 'to be on the safe side'. Calling a doctor in most cases was routine, to check the placenta, or to have a look at the baby. The only real worry they had, Honor says, was the possibility that she might haemorrhage. It is at this stage particularly, that problems can occur for the mother. The afterbirth, for example, has to come away whole and entire. If it does not, there is a danger that a woman may bleed more than she should. Four women out of the 15 had complications requiring medical assistance.

Cindy had to go to hospital the day after the birth:

I had a very small tear, but it was, like, it was on a vein. So I had to go to hospital the next day. It was just as well I did, because there was still a bit of the placenta inside. I had a D and C, and it was okay.

So did Ingrid. She haemorrhaged within a few hours of the birth:

> The problem was that the uterus was not contracting quickly enough. I have a slightly tilted uterus, and this is why I had the problem. At twelve o'clock, I felt really faint, and we decided to call the doctor. The bleeding had stopped by the time I went in.

By then she had lost a pint and a half of blood. It was what doctors would call 'a primary post-partum haemorrhage'. The doctors thought she had attempted an abortion: 'They didn't see the baby in his father's arms.' She received two blood transfusions. When she tried to arrange for her discharge, the doctor refused to speak to her: 'They don't talk to "hysterical women",' she says.

Una had a hard time releasing a large baby, who seemed to be stuck in gear for a while. Her husband called the doctor after it was all over: 'The bleeding was a bit too heavy. My blood pressure dropped. I was very cold.' Una was later diagnosed as anaemic.

Pamela's placenta did not detach itself cleanly from the womb:

> The afterbirth came away, but there were bits left. There was a bit of bleeding. The doctor palpitated it to make it come away.

Nor did her pubic bone fit back into place properly until much later.

༄

The Ethics of Unattended Birth

To some extent, the ethics of an unattended birth are the same as the ethics of any home birth which is professionally attended. Before going on to consider what has been described as the ultimate 'obstetrical horror', the birth that takes place unsupervised, let us look at the overlap, the area where the mother's right to choose is pitted against the baby's right to life. In his book, *Power and the Profession of Obstetrics*,[13] William Arney describes how in the United States, from the 1940s onwards, women posed a significant threat to the autonomy of obstetrics. After 1950, he says, obstetricians began to treat the fetus as a second patient, finding in the fetus 'not just a new point for intervening in pregnancy but also a way to blunt the critical edge of women's concerns about the way obstetricians treated them . . . Obstetricians could leave their treatment of the mother-to-be out of the debate entirely, for now they had the fetus'.

Have you the right to risk your baby's life, women planning an *attended* home birth are asked. According to obstetricians, the infant's need to be born in what they have defined as a safe environment, i.e. an obstetric unit, takes precedence over the mother's desire to give birth in what doctors have described as the *comfort* of her own home. It is a perspective that pits the baby's needs against those of the mother, setting 'overriding' physical needs against 'mere' psychological ones. It is rooted in the perception that the baby is a passenger in the carriage of its mother's body – the 'hard and soft passages', as they are called.[14] It is also rooted in the notion of the mind-body split, in the idea that the two are separate and function, somehow, independently of each other, just like the passenger and the passages. While women may speak about 'carrying' babies, they do not see themselves as 'carriers', any more than they regard their babies as 'parasites' in the 'maternal environment'. If you see your baby as part of you, there can be no conflict of interests between you.[15]

The trouble with risk is that, in addition to being a reality, it is also a perception. Separating the reality from the perception is impossible. If you believe in natural childbirth, you may believe that the management of birth in hospital is potentially hazardous. You may believe that it is safer to have a baby at home, where you can be certain that labour will not be artificially brought on or speeded up, before the baby is ready to be born. You may feel less at risk in an environment where no dangerous drugs can possibly be forced on you, nor any technology used which could lead to an unnecessary Caesarian section.

As Brian Spurrett, the Australian obstetrician, has pointed out, there is no such thing as zero risk in childbirth.[16] In addition to the core risks (or what would have happened anyway, wherever the birth took place), each environment carries its own particular hazards. In hospital, to take one example, the risk of cross-infection is infinitely greater than it is at home. At home, the risk may lie in the fact that it is a two-hour drive to hospital. But like apples and oranges, these risks are not comparable. And as Brian Spurrett admits, we have no way at present of measuring, statistically, what they are. Nor, he might have added, are we likely to in the future.

If mind and body are not separate, but interdependent,[17] then your feelings matter as much as the size and shape of your pelvis. You may feel that your labour will be easier if you are relaxed. You may feel that the baby's physical safety depends on your emotional well-being,[18] that the stress of going to hospital might lead to complications that could be avoided by staying at home. And if you do not see birth as a pathology, as a sign of disease, you may consider home to be a more appropriate place.

If you look at birth from the baby's point of view, a 'gentle' birth may be a priority. You may feel bound to give birth at home for the sake of the baby's future well-being. If you believe that unbroken physical contact during the first hours and days after birth is critical, then you may see home as the only place for bonding. And if you see birth as a family event, involving your partner and your other children, then home may appear best for everyone.

The notion of what is moral is rooted in free will, in our

ability to choose. And the choices we make depend on what we perceive as good and on what appears to be of most benefit to ourselves and to others.

Fíona recalled how in a hospital antenatal clinic she was told that having a child at home was dangerous. They made her feel guilty, and that she was pandering to herself. Selfishness may be the most hurtful accusation we can hurl at mothers, as Barbara Katz Rothman has pointed out.[19] To be a 'good' mother is to be 'unselfish'. There is this idea, she says, that women's needs are not important. In place of this, she reminds us that there is an alternative approach, one that recognizes women's autonomy and women's right to a quality of life.

How much sacrifice can we demand of a woman, Barbara Katz Rothman asks, albeit in another context. Even if you do not have any strong views on the way childbirth should be handled, you may still object to the way it is done in hospital. You may see hospital treatment as impersonal, humiliating, and degrading. You may feel certain procedures make labour more difficult and more painful to endure. For some women, birth in hospital *is* frightening. And the possibility that women may be more vulnerable to postnatal depression in hospital is never taken into account in the medical calculation of 'risk'.

If women are more than simply hard and soft passages, mere carriers of 'passengers', then free will enters into the equation. Controlling your own life, making your own choices, becomes important. You may equate taking responsibility for your own health, for your own body, with being an adult. If you see hospital as a place where you are not allowed to do this, you may regard it as more responsible to give birth elsewhere. You may see it as necessary to give birth in an environment where you have a measure of control over what is happening, where you are not handing over your body, where you are not giving up your responsibility for the birth of your baby.

The risks of home birth are either absolute or relative. If the risks are relative, as the maternity services in the Netherlands show,[20] then the argument shifts. It becomes an argument over the quality of the service. Home birth cannot be safe in one country and dangerous in another.

In the United States, the legal status of midwives varies enormously. In some states, independent professional practice is outlawed; in others lay midwifery is licensed.[21] In Britain, there was a furore some years ago when fathers were prosecuted for illegal midwifery.[22] After Una had given birth, the public health nurse told her that it was illegal to have a home birth. Several fathers asked about the law on unattended birth in Ireland. Although the Nurses' Act (1985) prohibits unqualified persons from attending a woman in childbirth, no prosecutions have ever been brought. The Act allows for attendance in childbirth, other than for reward, 'in cases of sudden or urgent necessity where neither a midwife nor a registered medical practitioner is immediately available'.[23]

When the state refuses to provide a maternity service at home, women – some women – will have unattended births. In the larger group, women who managed to get a midwife or a doctor were asked whether they would have considered delivering the baby themselves, had they not been able to get professional help. As many as 19 per cent said they would consider going it alone. If we were to jail people for dying at home, if we were to institutionalize death in the same way that we have institutionalized birth, there would be an outcry. If we attempt to compel women to give birth in hospital, there are no lengths to which they will not go. Unattended birth must carry an additional margin of risk. It is a risk, however, which some women are prepared to take.

☙ 8 ☙

Motherhood and Doctorhood

Birth is part of life. Not only in the mystical sense, but also because it belongs to the here and now. How you deal with it depends on who you are. How you see it depends on how you see yourself, on how you see the world and your place in it.

Do women choosing home delivery see birth as a fact of life or as a voyage of discovery? Is home birth just an isolated issue for women, or is it part and parcel of a moving away from medicine as we know it? How does home birth relate to feminism? Such questions all centre on the main issue: can a consensus be reached among women on birth?

☙

Thinking About Birth

The way we look at birth has changed profoundly over the past fifty years. Women are having far fewer children, for one thing. And, as the experience has become rarer, so its value has increased. In her introduction to *Birth at Home*,[1] Sheila Kitzinger summarizes her view of how women today see birth: there is an emphasis on nature; on the couple ('birth as a high point in the rhythm of their lives together'); and lastly, there is the symbolic significance of birth, encompassing the idea of rebirth, and, ultimately, the recreation of the human spirit.

Control over fertility has changed the signification of birth.

Having a child is no longer inevitable. Within the group, many women regard birth as an event, an experience, not unlike sex in its physical intimacy, which they invest with emotion and with meaning. For some, there is the perception of birth as a climax after the months of pregnancy, as a voyage into the interior of the self. Lucinda wanted to do it on her own, without drugs, to find out what was there:

> You go into an inner state. It's almost like leaving the earth. It's the effect of the hormones on the body. What's happening in your body takes over your mind. They are natural forces. You find out how powerful they are.

For Hilary, there is a similar blurring of the boundaries between the inner and the outer world:

> It is a time when you are able to transcend yourself, when you can take in so much more, when you can feel at one with the world. The moment of birth is very sacred. It is one moment in our lives when we are really in touch with ourselves. It can't be repeated.

Death, and birth, are both part of the life process. Birth, Rosemary says, made her realize 'how delicate, and yet how strong life is. I felt privileged to be able to participate in it.' Other women also display this same reverence for life. Birth is an act of creation. You are producing life, women say. But what is life? How you perceive birth depends, to a degree, on how you see life.

For some women, giving birth is more than bringing a body of flesh and blood into the world. For some women, the body *is* the spirit made flesh. For Roman Catholics, as for others, the soul is created at the moment of conception. Thea believes, not in the Catholic doctrine of ensoulment, but in the idea of a prior existence, a spiritual life before birth. Babies choose to be born in a certain atmosphere, she says, in a particular environment:

> The spirit needs a chance to incarnate. At birth, the spirit

is hardly in this world, in this body. We have lessons to learn in our lives. The spirit dresses itself in a certain body to learn.

For Beatrix, too, there is this sense of predestination, a working-out of what has been ordained:

> I believe in astral bodies, the other body, the one where the emotions are. I believe that children choose their parents. I believe in reincarnation. We have all known each other in past lives. The children have to play their part in this life. They do this by choosing us.

Incarnation, reincarnation, past lives, future lives: seen in this eternal light, birth assumes boundless and unimaginable significance. The arrival of this infant trailing clouds of glory from another world, the moment of incarnation, becomes sacred, finite and infinite, all at once.

Asked about their religious beliefs, 14 per cent of the group define themselves as *spiritual*, although they have no formal faith or creed. It is important to allow birth its spiritual side, Virginia explains, 'to give it that wholeness'. She had arranged for a friend, a midwife in England who is a Buddhist nun, to deliver her baby:

> We played classical music. There was a warm fire and we burned incense. We made a Buddhist shrine in the house. She asked me if she could bless the baby, and that fitted in with our ideas of what birth is about. Birth . . . is under-expressed as a ceremony.

Women like Virginia see home as offering greater freedom to define birth as a spiritual event. Their sense of the spiritual forms part of the background to their decision to have a home birth. Neither these women, nor their partners would allow birth to be profaned in hospital.

They are, undoubtedly, in a minority. A third of the group say they have no religious beliefs of any kind. Another third are Roman Catholic. Despite the doctrine of ensoulment, Catholic women saw no connection between their religious beliefs and their decision to have a baby at home.

In the United States, home birth is associated with fundamentalism, and with religious groups who practise alternative healing.[2] Hardly anyone within this group held fundamentalist beliefs. Muslims, evangelical Christians, Mormons and Jehovah's Witnesses accounted for only seven per cent of the group. Moreover, these women were not necessarily fundamentalist in their beliefs. The only Jehovah's Witness in the group says she was afraid they might force a blood transfusion on her in hospital. Yet, the connection between religious beliefs and home birth was rarely as direct as this.

There is a belief that the general atmosphere around a child at the moment of birth is very important. The spiritual atmosphere comes from the energy of those present, Ursula maintains. Some women believe that the experience of birth imprints itself on the mind, and that birth affects the development of the personality. Trudi maintains that 'The time of birth is very important, and the way you are born.' Astrology is based on this belief. In the commune Trudi grew up in, they used hypnosis and visualization to re-live the moment of birth. Birth was seen as the primary welcome into the world. It is vitally important, according to Ursula, 'to have that support, love and bliss from the beginning'. Like a few others in the group, she believes in rebirthing, a New Age therapy aimed at unlocking the moment of birth, thereby releasing negative thought patterns and feelings that have built up over the years.[3] Women who believe in rebirthing talk about the need to be born in an atmosphere of love rather than fear.

The power women attribute to birth is both positive and negative. There is only one birth for each baby, Fionnuala says, emphasizing the irrevocable and unalterable nature of the event. On the positive side, there is the idea of birth as growth. Ute says her greatest fear would be to have a Caesarian section, because it would deprive the baby of the experience of being born: 'It is part of a full life to experience birth. Children need to have the experience of birth in order to find their way in the world.' On the negative side, there is the belief that a difficult birth can damage the baby,[4] the conviction that if the birth is not gentle, then the baby may see the world as harsh and unwelcoming. The birthing process should be calmer, Delma says: 'It would prevent psychological problems later. Babies are traumatized.'

If birth is about life, it is also indissociable from motherhood.[5] For a husband and wife, Frances says, birth is a fulfilment:

> It is what fulfils a marriage . . . Home is the way to have your baby . . . The children are our priority . . . To be a good mother comes before everything else. I believe in the natural process.

The idea that the birth of children fulfils a marriage is to be found in the words of the Roman Catholic marriage service, but the religious emphasis on procreation is universal. Mary elevates motherhood to a near-mystical plane:

> The way birth is allowed to take place is fundamental to society. That life starts at the very beginning in the proper way. Hospital takes away the motherhood.

If there is no agreement as to the meaning of birth, as to the significance of life, there is one aspect of labour on which there is a consensus. Hilary speaks for the great majority of women when she says: 'The way you are dealt with in birth affects your baby. It affects the way you think about your baby, the way you think about yourself.' In hospital, Deborah says, their priority is healthy babies, implying that their priorities are too narrow. They should have due regard for the emotional health of the mother, she feels. If birth has the power to affect your self-esteem, and your relationships, women conclude, it should be more personal and less technical.

The traditional view of childbirth tends to reduce rather than increase its significance. Mona's view is nothing if not matter-of-fact: 'Having a baby at home is just another job in the house,' she says. The traditional view is a minority one, held by one-fifth of the group. Lucinda describes how she was telling one woman later about her experience, and the woman responded by saying, 'You dirty thing!' Deirdre describes birth as 'general unpleasantness':

> The whole procedure is not pleasant. When I think of the job binmen have, and people cleaning out sewers, and I think of what midwives have to do – it's an awful job.[6]

This idea of birth as 'dirty' can be traced back to religion, for example, to the Jansenist belief in the body as unclean. Christianity required new mothers to purify themselves by submitting to a religious ceremony known as 'churching'. Sheila Kitzinger shows that, in traditional cultures, ceremonies of cleansing and purification following the segregation of mother and child after birth were central to childbirth rituals all over the world.[7] In Europe, gypsy culture demands that a new mother be given her own tent and crockery; both tent and bedding are ritually burned at the end of the period of seclusion. In Japan in the seventeenth century, a woman was secluded for thirty-five days following childbirth. Today, she is still prohibited from visiting a shrine during this period.

But most of all, it is Deirdre's insistence that birth is of no importance that is the hallmark of traditional thinking: 'Birth at home is a non-event – it doesn't disturb the household . . . It's part of life.' Here, 'life' is matter-of-fact, down to earth and temporal, not cosmic, boundless and eternal. Here, life is something you just get on with.

༄

Back to Nature

Home birth fitted in. We're vegetarian, slightly alternative. I believe in a natural way of doing things [Angela].

Home birth is part of an overall attitude to life, Statia's husband maintains, part of self-sufficiency. 'When we moved down here, it was pioneering,' Lorna says: 'We were growing our own vegetables, making our own beer and wine.' Statia and her husband are urban refugees, who sold up and went to live on a small-holding in the green world. For some, home birth, along with homesteading and homeschooling, is a move away from the institutions of the state. It is an expression of other ideas, other values. In Ireland, home birth is linked to deschooling, to environmental groups and co-operative movements of all kinds. For some – if not for all – home birth forms part of a wider opposition to the way society is organized. Asked for their political views, 10 per cent of women in the group described themselves as Green.

However, alongside the women who declared an interest in spirituality, Greens were a minority within the group. Over half of the group maintained that they had no political views one way or another. Many of the women were highly critical of the political process. Some were cynical, others were alienated. Many said that they had no interest in politics. Interestingly, only four per cent of the women described themselves, politically, as conservative.

৵

Natural Childbirth: The Great Debate

In our personal belief systems, we integrate different values, different ideas. For Jacqueline, a Muslim, there is a direct link between her personal faith in God and her belief that birth should be natural: 'Anything that is natural is related to faith – the more natural, the nearer to God.' For over two-thirds of the group, their belief in natural childbirth was central to their decision to have a home birth (see Chapter 3). Niamh could not understand why she had to go to hospital to have a baby:

I was so used to my father having all these animals around

at home. If the cow can have a calf, the dog pups, and the cat kittens . . . I reckon there's nobody likely to carry a baby who can't deliver that baby.

The view that pregnancy and birth are 'natural' seems to assume that 'nature' is inherently 'good'. Like Grantly Dick-Read,[8] Fionnuala talks about the effects of 'civilization' on labour:

In cultures where birth is expected to be easy, then it's easy. In cultures where it's expected to lead to complications, then that's what happens.

The women in the tribes have no pain, Katherina says. However, Ann Oakley has pointed out that when women appeal to 'nature' in support of their wish to avoid medical intervention in labour, they may well be alluding to the more basic issue of control over birth.[9] Only in retrospect, obstetricians say, can labour be seen to be normal. The idea of pregnancy as a disease was reinforced by the idea that the safety of birth depended on attendance by doctors.[10] Within the group, women refuse to see themselves as ill just because they are pregnant, and they see hospital as an alien environment. It is an unnecessary hardship, Hilary maintains, to have to go to hospital: 'You're surrounded by medical instruments, clanging silver, stainless steel, in a sterile atmosphere.'

Many women feel that having to move in labour to get to the hospital appointed for their delivery is unnatural and hazardous. Nobody would move a cow in labour unless they really had to, Nora says. (Again, the appeal to 'nature', to what happens naturally in the animal kingdom.) Many women talk about how artificial it is to have to go away, to leave your own environment. You have to adjust to your surroundings, Statia explains, then you have to readjust again when you come home: 'The natural processes of the body should be allowed.' Finally, in this alien environment, there is the danger of infection to the baby.

Many women believe the tension caused by being in hospital is in itself a risk, that medical procedures create a situation which leads to more complications. If you are worried, they say, it affects your labour.[11] Some women see illness as psychosomatic, believing that physical illness or disease can originate in the mind. Other women reject the idea that one can divide the mind from the body at all.[12] In attributing complications in labour to emotional factors, for instance, women part company with doctors, who treat the body as though it were a machine.[13] Pain, for example, is seen by obstetricians as a physiological response to the 'stimulus' of labour.[14] Women, however, report an inverse relationship between pain and autonomy: the less control they have over the event, the more pain they say they experience.

Susan, a nurse, singles out some of the hospital routines women find distressing:

> Fatima Hospital is still very, very ritualized. They still give you an enema and a full shave. It only introduces infection. You are still tied to the bed. If you want to walk around, you can't. There isn't room. You can't even have a cup of tea.

Fatima is a teaching hospital. Not wanting to be 'tied to the bed' in labour is one thing: believing that it is counterproductive is another. Ursula, an independent antenatal teacher, believes that it is very important to be upright and to be moving around: 'Studies have been done which show that there is a longer gap between the contractions, and that they are more *efficient*,' she says.[15]

Lucinda believes that doing an internal can also be counterproductive:

> When I went in first, they did an internal. That slowed down the labour. The wave pattern of the contractions, it's like some kind of electrical energy. If you interfere with it, you stop it. I read about it afterwards.

Women who believe in natural childbirth tend to belong to the birth organizations, and to read books on birth. If natural childbirth started out as 'childbirth without fear', before becoming 'prepared childbirth', with women working hand in glove with doctors in hospital,[16] it is now becoming nothing less than a revolt against the way obstetricians manage birth in hospital. Statia believes they treat birth as though it were inherently abnormal. The net result of all of this management, she says, is 'total lack of control for women'. Like other women who believe in natural childbirth, Cecilia resents the way that birth is treated as a pathology: 'If pregnancy and birth are a disease, then the cure is high-tech equipment.' There is a suspicion that hospital procedures are for the convenience of the hospital, not for the welfare of the patient. In hospital, Nuala says, disapprovingly, they can tell you when your baby is going to be born. 'They nearly push it out for you,' Rachel adds, sarcastically.

According to Aylish, a former midwife, it is counter-productive to shorten labour in a normal birth: 'You can cope better with a slightly more long-drawn-out labour than you can with a shorter, more intense one.'[17] Many women agree. They have these drips 'to *fasten* labour to suit themselves,' Chrissie observes. Shortening labour, as far as women can see, is a large part of what obstetrics is all about. In hospital, Lelia says, they create the situation that creates the problem:

One things leads to another. If they break the waters and that doesn't work, then they've got to do something else to get the labour going. It's the fact that there's just x amount of time in which to get that baby out, regardless.

Lelia identifies the core of the matter: time *is* of the essence. In hospital, every labour is plotted on a graph, based on what is known as 'Friedman's curve'. An American obstetrician, Emmanuel Friedman, developed a graph of the 'ideal' labour in the 1950s, plotting the dilatation of a woman's cervix against time. Since the baby's head is approximately 10 centimetres in diameter, and the maximum time allowed is 10 hours, the slowest rate of dilatation acceptable is one centimetre per hour.[18] Helena talks about being put 'under pressure to produce', about not wanting to be 'forced, cajoled, or coerced into unnecessary procedures'. However, since nature cannot be relied upon to produce a baby within this time, actively managing labour means that certain procedures may be called for. Sooner or later, on admission to the labour unit or after, the waters are broken. Within several hours, oxytocin, or more recently, prostaglandin, will be given to first-time mothers unless significant progress, defined as 'one notional centimetre', has been made.[19] A woman whose labour does not follow Friedman's curve may be diagnosed as suffering from 'dystocia', or 'failure to progress'. Caesarian sections are performed for 'failure to progress'.[20]

Catherine, who delivered two hundred babies as part of her midwifery training, explains how routine hospital procedures can cause complications:

> There's no need for all these internal examinations. One or two is enough, it introduces infection. I don't agree with mothers being in bed in labour. Lying in bed waiting for each contraction makes it more difficult. They don't let nature take its course. They put up drips. It's cruelty to bring on labour. Oxytocin makes it unbearable. I've seen them when they've taken pethidine. They lose control, dignity.

Rupturing the membranes routinely, according to Ursula, accelerates contractions and makes them more uncomfortable.[21] 'Stimulating' labour with oxytocin may make it necessary for women to take pethidine, a synthetic opiate. The authors of *Active Management of Labor* admit that oxytocin causes painful contractions 'whether or not a woman is in labour'.[22] Aylish maintains that if she had to have oxytocin, she would have an epidural.[23] Obstetric textbooks emphasize the need for drugs to relieve pain in labour; they also discuss at length the risks involved in the use of such drugs. Oxytocin is not without its dangers, Aylish points out: 'There is a slight risk of rupturing the womb. It is also associated with jaundice in the baby,' she maintains. Obstetricians accept that oxytocin can cause rupture of the womb in a second or subsequent pregnancy, but they dispute the association with jaundice in the baby, except where oxytocin is used to induce the birth.[24]

Avoiding drugs in labour, whether anaesthetic, analgesic or accelerating, is at the heart of natural childbirth.[25] Nora believes drugs make labour high-risk. On the subject of painkillers in labour, a World Health Organization report states that there is no question but that these drugs affect the unborn baby.[26] Aylish says that the amount of pethidine that is given is not enough to kill the pain, but it is enough to kill the baby:

> The amount of pethidine is supposed to be related to body weight, but in practice they give 50mg plus 50mg Sparine (a tranquillizer). It depresses the baby's respiratory centre. I had a friend who worked in Africa. She gave the mother pethidine, and the baby was born dead because of that. The mother went from three centimetres to ten, just like that. We have the antidote here, but she didn't. It was a bush hospital.

The drugged infant with a depressed respiratory system and depressed brain is well documented in the medical literature. Women who believe in natural childbirth are well acquainted with the spectre of the baby whose breathing is impaired by drugs (see Chapter 3). The most frequent argument they put forward against pethidine is that it is harmful to the baby. The placenta used to be thought of as a barrier, impervious to everything. Women now know that drugs in labour cross the placenta. Pethidine interferes with bonding and with feeding, Aylish believes: 'They say it makes the baby dopey for a couple of days. Babies should be very alert when they are born.'

The techniques used to accelerate labour are also used to induce it. In the late 1960s and early 1970s, induction rates skyrocketed in Britain,[27] and in other European countries.[28] Unlike acceleration, induction has been widely censured. There was public outrage in the wake of a 1976 BBC documentary which cast doubt on the safety of current obstetric practices, such as inducing labour.[29] Over the next few years, induction rates fell in British Maternity Hospitals. Although social or convenience induction became more difficult to justify, the practice of routinely inducing labour once pregnancy has gone so many days over the 'estimated date of delivery' is still standard in many hospitals. Susan explains what happens in Fatima Hospital:

> If you're ten days overdue, that's it. You're induced. But they have the technology now. With blood tests, they can tell whether or not the placenta is adequate.

Induction, Ursula suggests, means that painkillers become necessary. Labour is induced in precisely the same way that it is speeded up, by breaking the waters, and by means of oxytocin or prostaglandin. The only difference, and it is a substantial one, particularly for the baby, is that inducing labour terminates the pregnancy artificially, exposing the baby to the potential hazards of a premature birth. In some hospitals, twin pregnancies are routinely induced, and induction rates of 20 per cent or more for first-time mothers are standard.[30]

Induction is associated with increased rates of prematurity, fetal distress, jaundice, and infections in the mother.[31] It is linked with more pain, with greater use of painkillers, and with higher rates[32] of forceps, vacuum and Caesarian deliveries.[33] Induction, the WHO says, may be a crucial step in an interlocking chain of intervention, with one medical procedure increasing the likelihood that further medical treatment will be necessary.[34]

Continuous fetal monitoring is another link in the same chain. Harriet says women have been hoodwinked into thinking that they should rely more on machines:

> Women are told that what they know about their bodies is less than what the machine knows. This leads to fear, which creates tension, which leads to difficult births.

The machine to which Harriet refers is the electronic fetal monitor, which has been described as the most controversial innovation in obstetrics since the introduction of the forceps in the seventeenth century.[35] Continuous fetal monitoring used to be reserved for high-risk labours; now in some hospitals it is for everyone. It is all done for the sake of the hospital system, Tara says, like social induction or the drip in labour. Women see routine monitoring as unnecessary and even harmful. Monitoring puts pressure on you, they say, to produce. Only 5 per cent of deliveries are complicated, Statia maintains, but the other 95 per cent are managed in the same way, with the same technology. Biddy believes that the birth machines are eroding midwifery skills: 'I think they are losing hands-on diagnosis.' Hilda takes this argument even further: 'Midwives are losing their autonomy, and becoming only obstetrical nurses.'

Monitoring can be external or it can be internal, and this kind of physically invasive monitoring is becoming standard.[36] Electronic fetal monitoring (EFM) confines women to bed during labour, bringing back a hospital routine that had been abandoned to some extent, and one to which women object.

The risk of infection in EFM has been well established in a number of studies.[37] The artificial breaking of the waters which it entails represents a risk of infection to the baby. In addition, attaching a clip to the baby's scalp can cause a small break or wound in the baby's skin. There is also a risk of infection to the woman.

Electronic fetal monitoring is automatic. How to listen to the fetal heart is no longer a problem; what to listen for is another matter. Some fetal heart patterns are believed by obstetricians to be ominous; others continue to be a matter of dispute.[38] Reading fetal distress where there is none is known as a 'false positive' reading. Where fetal distress is suspected, the medical response is to deliver the baby swiftly.

Rose, a nurse, sees hospital practice and procedure as stemming from a fear of litigation. They want the baby out as quickly as possible, she says: 'It's a kind of hysteria.' Continuous monitoring, Geraldine adds, leads to a kind of paranoia. She talks about the rise in the number of emergency Caesarian sections, done for fear of litigation: 'We are seeing defensive medicine.'[39] Electronic fetal monitoring has been partly responsible for a dramatic increase in Caesarian sections in many countries.[40] Some obstetricians would dispute this; others would argue in favour of expanding the 'indications' for Caesarian, given the operation's increased safety.[41] What is beyond dispute is that monitoring is lucrative. As far back as 1978, the total US market was worth over $30 million. In one year alone in Britain, one electronics firm sold over 800 monitors for more than two million pounds. Whether or not perinatal outcomes – death and sickness rates – are improved by monitoring is unproven.[42]

Women respond to this plethora of procedures, drugs, and machines by opting for epidurals. The epidural is a new link in an old chain, linking anaesthetics to obstetrics.[43] People should be given more information, Fionnuala believes: 'If a woman wants an epidural, she's not told it's a package. You may not have forceps, but it is more likely.' Her labour is now deemed to need more intensive care, and in some hospitals, EFM is part of the package. Since she cannot now control her bladder, a catheter is needed.[44] Inserting a catheter carries some risk of infection, and there is also a slight possibility of damage to the urethra. Stress incontinence has also come up as a possible consequence, but the jury is still out on this, as on other after-childbirth complaints reported by women[45] such as headaches, other aches and pains and haemorrhoids.

The verdict is beginning to come in, however, on the possibility that birth by epidural may lead to serious long-term back trouble. 'Post-epidural back pain' has now become a recognized category in anaesthetic research. According to Christine MacArthur's study, having an epidural may double the risk: one woman in five may be affected, and this is almost double the rate for women who labour without an epidural. She may suffer from what anaesthetists call 'chronic non-malignant pain', which may be bad enough to warrant surgery.[46]

Doris Haire, an American author widely read by women,

suggests that there may be other risks. Arguing against the use of both painkilling and anaesthetic drugs in labour, she says that in addition to their short-term effects, these drugs, by penetrating the baby's central nervous system expose him to possible long-term neurological damage.[47]

These risks – stress incontinence for example, or neurological damage in babies[48] – are unproven, and partly because they are long-term, they may continue to be so. Real or imaginary,[49] these are the risks of the epidural that works as it should. If the epidural needle does not go into what is called the 'epidural space' around the spinal cord, then a woman may be paralysed or worse.[50, 51] Statistically, the risk of paralysis or death is very, very small: in practice, because it is inherent in the procedure itself, the actual risk depends on the skill and experience of the anaesthetist involved. For many obstetricians, the salient risk is the risk of operative delivery. Obstetricians acknowledge that the use of a Kjellands or high forceps, for example, represents a serious risk to the mother and to the baby.[52] The proportion of forceps deliveries which can be attributed to epidurals is hotly debated. In the absence of research, hospital statistics and clinical estimates are all we have to go on. An overall rate of one in three has been recorded,[53] while for first-time mothers, rates of 40–60 per cent have been quoted.[54] Anaesthetists tend towards the positive view that epidurals do not increase the number of deliveries performed by operation.[55] However, according to Dr Frederick Frigoletto, head of obstetrics at Harvard Medical School, having an epidural multiplies by four the risk of Caesarian section for 'low-risk' women.[56]

࿎

Nature, Health and Drug Therapy

If home birth is an expression of natural childbirth, it is also related to women's views on health care, generally. Women's belief in natural childbirth is rooted in their opposition to the use of drugs in labour.[57] For some women, this is part of a wider opposition to what they see as the overuse of drugs by general practitioners. There is not enough attention paid to diet, or to the environment, women feel. Or to the emotions. Katherina evokes memories of a golden age when she was young in Germany: 'The family doctor knew all about herbs. He would advise you on diet, he would use poultices.' Many women, like Charlotte, simply refuse to take prescribed drugs: 'I will go to a doctor for diagnosis but I prefer not to take anything . . . No aspirins, no vaccinations, no antibiotics.'

The drug companies, in Biddy's view, have practically taken over from the medical profession:

> Notebooks, leaflets, notepads, they're all from pharmaceutical companies. The drug companies are almost telling the doctor what the symptoms are, [what drug to use], what the dosage is, what the side-effects are. It lessens their doctorhood.

As Mary sees it, doctors may well allow themselves to be influenced by drug companies in their choice of drugs. She talks about the money spent by companies in promoting new drugs: 'A new list comes out every year from the drug companies . . . The doctors get big perks from the drug companies if they prescribe their products.' She sees the industry as being dangerously out of control: 'They are trying out drugs that haven't even been tested.'

It is all money, obstetricians, machines and drug companies, Tríona maintains, describing what she sees as the birth industry. Jo gives one example of what she feels is the costly waste of resources in an expanding market: 'Lots of money is spent on comprehensive screening – of healthy women having healthy pregnancies.' Routine ultrasound scanning, according to the WHO, is of no benefit.[58] Catherine, whose father is a doctor, has a particularly harsh view of the system: 'Maternity hospitals are appalling, money-making machines.' Frances, a former nurse, believes that consultants have a vested interest in maintaining birth in hospital: 'Doctors are anti-home birth – it's financial.' She is not alone in this view.

Sometimes it is difficult to know whether women are generalizing from their birth experiences to medicine as a whole or whether their views on health care shaped their opinions of maternity care.

In the United States, at least $10 billion is spent annually on alternative health care.[59] It is not so much that women who choose home birth are believers in what the late Trinity College lecturer, Petr Skrabanek, called 'sympathetic magic'.[60] It is more that, like Linda, they have lost their faith in orthodox medicine:

> Doctors treat symptoms now. There is no real doctoring . . . They should take a more personal interest. There is too much emphasis on drugs. The younger the doctor, the worse he is.

Only four per cent of women express satisfaction with medicine as we know it. Asked about their treatment preferences, one third of the group show a preference for some form of alternative treatment. Homeopathy emerges as the single most widely used form of alternative medicine, with acupuncture in second place. A small number of women had consulted alternative practitioners, such as osteopaths, and their traditional Irish counterparts, bone-setters. In Ireland, alternative medicine ranges from New Age therapists to traditional healers. Women consulted chiropractors, spinologists and allergists; they also went to herbalists and faith healers. To treat illness, Ursula says she would use 'rebirthing, massage, acupressure, homeopathy, spiritual healing, or reflexology'. Rachel says she relies upon cures: 'Of course, if you went to the doctor, you wouldn't tell him. And you wouldn't tell the cure you'd been to the doctor.' Like many other women, Harriet makes it clear that she would prefer to deal with a health problem herself:

> Through nursing, through giving the child the best available food, through vitamins, through holding the child,

through working out how it happened. For me it's a question of diet, understanding and nursing.

Diet is an aspect of health which women feel is ignored by doctors. As far as they are concerned, doctors have neither interest nor training in nutrition. Dympna links the question of nutrition with a controversial issue, namely, vaccinations:

> Vaccinations damage the liver and the immune system . . .
> Alternative nutritionalists believe that if the diet is healthy, they will take these diseases in their stride.

This is a minority view within the group. The majority of mothers had their children immunized, and reflecting the spectrum of views on the topic, 15 per cent did not vaccinate their children at all. This opposition to vaccinations from women choosing home birth is part of a wider trend, as American studies show.[61] Women have different reasons for refusing to have their children immunized. During the first two years, Katherina says, children do not need vaccinations:

> I believe in God. If they are to get it, they will get it. Vaccinations do harm. They weaken the child. For the first seven years, they incarnate.

Incarnation, or ensoulment, is the incorporation of the soul into the body, which begins, according to Katherina, at the moment of birth. There are women who believe that childhood illnesses are a necessary part of growth and development. Underlying their opposition to mass immunization programmes are positive ideas of child development, of physical and even spiritual, growth.

Geraldine does not believe, either, in immunizing against whooping cough, mumps, or measles:

> They are childhood illnesses. They are part of the development of the child. We damage the immune system by injecting these things into the bloodstream.

248

Nearly every woman in the group who refused to have her child immunized believes that vaccinations lower the child's resistance by damaging the immune system. Catherine believes immunizations can cause a child's growth to be retarded: 'Vaccinations are quite dangerous for young kids. Exposing young children to even minimal doses can cause slight impairments in growth.' Vaccinations are affecting the underlying immunity of the herd, Geraldine claims: 'Ireland has the highest rates of Alzheimer's disease in the world, with the exception of Israel. And we have the highest vaccination levels.'[62] Finally, there is the knowledge that the health industry is being driven by market forces: 'There is huge money being made out of it.'

As many as 34 per cent of women feel that general practitioners take an artificially restricted and overly narrow view of health; they see medical diagnosis as being based on fragments of their physical selves, the piecing together of isolated symptoms, without reference to the person as a whole. Geraldine is scathing in her criticism of general practice: 'General practitioners don't deal with the cause, they deal with the symptoms. They give out Dozol like it was lemonade.' Regular medicine does not get to the root of things, according to Delma: 'The mind and the body, both are fused. You can't say which comes first'.[63] Niamh says she had an aunt who used to rattle like a pill-box:

> Doctors don't get to the bottom of things – they're doling out Valium for depression. They should have more time to talk, to listen to people.

Doctors only see the physical signs of disease, according to Tríona:

> They look at the lungs, or the liver, or whatever. They do not see that the physical outcomes of people are the result of spiritual and emotional disorders.

When women accuse doctors of not being holistic in their

approach to health, of not getting to the root of the problem, it is because they see the root of illness as emotional. The idea of the mind-body split is a rather old idea, attributed to the seventeenth-century French philosopher, Descartes. Far from having been discarded as dated or useless, it is an idea that forms the foundation of modern Western medicine as we know it.[64]

A number of women feel that doctors only tell their patients what *they* think they should know. One third of the group are of the opinion that family doctors do not listen to their patients, and, in particular, to their women patients. Nearly as many feel that doctors are unwilling to allow people to exercise their autonomy, to make informed decisions on their care.

The wish to assume personal responsibility for the birth of one's baby, as often as not, forms part of a wider stance *vis-à-vis* health in general. For many women, there has been a shift in their understanding of what constitutes health, in their concept of illness, and how it should be treated. According to Rachel, they have taken away women's instinct to give birth. Women are reassessing the place of medicine in their lives. They are redefining the doctor's role. The notion of autonomy, the right to reserve to yourself the power to decide, is at the core of this shift in attitude. It underpins both the alternative health and the women's health movements:[65]

> I mistrust doctors. They treat the person like a bit of machinery. They feel they must take over, but the patient has a role in getting better [Rachel].

Rosemary sees people as wanting to be looked after. The doctor is perceived as a caring person in our society:

> When a doctor gives out drugs, he is seen to be doing something. Drugs are an extension of the role of carer. People don't want the responsibility of looking after their own health. They are very dependent. Western medicine is control-oriented, power-oriented.

If people fail to take responsibility for their health, Tríona believes, it is also because they are being targeted by an ever-expanding health industry:

> The effect of the health industry is that more and more people are classified as sick. But people have abdicated responsibility for their health. Problems arise from ignoring the mind and the soul.

Tríona's thinking is reminiscent of Ivan Illich's; his book *Limits to Medicine*[66] contains a chapter on the industrialization of death:

> Birth is part of life, like death. It's getting to the stage where you're not allowed to die except in hospital. Where you're not allowed to be born except in hospital . . . I'm a radical. I think we should get back to the roots.

Virginia also believes we are being denied the experience of birth and death in our society. They should be brought back into the community, Statia's husband says. 'You must have control over your own body, over your own health,' Patricia concludes: 'You're the one who knows most about it.'

∼

Our Bodies, Ourselves

> Home birth is related to my views on women – birth should not be taken away from them. You lose something when your responsibility has been taken away from you [Sarah, a former nurse].

It is your responsibility to govern your own labour, Catherine says: 'Doctors treat their advice as if it were God-given.' Birth belongs to women and they should reclaim it, Rosemary feels. Many women agree. Half of the group believe that childbirth has been overly medicalized, that doctors have taken over from women. One of the driving forces behind home birth since the late 1970s has been the women's health movement. Books like the Boston Women's Health Book Collective's, *Our Bodies, Ourselves*,[67] contain the idea that women need to reclaim their bodies, to take responsibility for their own health. It is an idea that has taken root in the minds of women everywhere.

Birth is part of women's rights, Hilary believes: 'Birth is being taken over, being taken out of their hands.' Opposing the idea of medical control over women's reproductive health, feminism, like alternative health, promotes instead ideas of self-reliance and self-determination. Hilda sees birth as a feminist issue: 'It is an individual woman's right to decide what happens to her body.' The right to own your own body is an idea that, for women, leads inevitably to childbirth. However, it brings women into conflict with doctors.

In obstetric textbooks, the baby is simply a passenger in the human carrier which is its mother.[68] Women do not see themselves as carriers. Rosemary talks about the attitude in hospital, which she sums up as 'We deliver your child'. It is a shame, Maeve says, that women are conditioned to think that birth is outside themselves: 'The doctor delivers the baby, this is what is said.' Nuala believes that women should be encouraged to have more confidence in themselves, that they should not be led into thinking that birth is like an operation.

Women with a more traditional view of birth see themselves as 'helping the doctor'. Within the group, they are in a minority. Many women are opposed to this idea, whether they express it as gender perception, or as feminist analysis. Having a home birth enhanced her sense of herself as a feminist, Sue feels:

> I saw my feminism as coming from a sense of well-being from being a woman, and doing this wonderful thing . . . I felt that this was what women should be striving for.

Asked for their political views, 28 per cent of women reply that they are feminists. They are women whose analysis of the world, of society in general, and of their own lives in particular, is gender-based. Rose, a former nurse, finds the male domination of childbirth irksome. She resented the idea that a group of men could dictate to women the place of birth: 'They were in hospital, so that's where you had to go.' Hilda, who has a background in theoretical physics, angrily sums up what she sees as the prevailing attitude in hospital: 'Now you just be a good little woman, and leave it to me, and everything will be all right.' There is a point in women's minds where obstetric control of labour and birth merges with male power over a female function.[69] Nadine, a Muslim, sees women's liberation as closely related to freedom in birth:

> Doctors wield so much power over birth ... Childbirth is very personal to me – I don't see why men should have control over it, which is what happens in hospitals.

Obstetricians, more often than not, are male.[70] For Aileen, there is the same blurring of the lines:

> Home birth is to do with the dignity of women. There are a lot of male doctors who don't understand where women are at ... Doctors don't see how significant women's feelings are.

Obstetrics is dominated by men, Ruth maintains: 'You can't run labour according to schedule. It is a typically male attitude.' Cassie is one of the few to have had a birth by epidural, complete with forceps. The effect of the epidural, she says, is that 'Someone else is in control. Someone else is taking over your body.' Taking drugs, according to Biddy, is crossing the border from being the one who gives birth to being the one whose baby is delivered. In this scenario, the woman has finally become an integral part of the process of production and any notions she may have had of control are redundant. In hospital, women say, birth is just a procedure. Cassie's argument against the epidural is similar to Rosemary's argument against pethidine. Birth should not be a managed experience, Rosemary feels:

> Drugs distort your perception. They interfere with your concentration. If you take pethidine, your mind is up there. It is meant to dissociate you from the pain.

Rosemary's belief in natural childbirth is reinforced by a feminist view of the world. There are opiates produced spontaneously by the body, she says: 'It doesn't need to be drug-managed. The body copes beautifully.' Pethidine she describes in gender terms as an 'unnecessary male-dominated procedure': 'Men think, "We'll give you something to get rid of the pain", but it's constructive pain.' She has identified an important difference in attitude towards pain in labour between doctors and women.[71] (Again, her words reflect her view of medical control as a form of male supremacy.) To Tríona also, the medical response to pain – to control it – is a male attitude: 'Men are trained not to allow pain. They can't see it as productive.' Geraldine develops this link between doing it yourself and doing without drugs, echoing Rosemary's belief in nature:

> I believe in self-reliance in health matters. I don't think in terms of painkillers. I wouldn't use acupuncture, for example [in labour]. If you have an epidural, you don't have this feeling that you're doing it yourself. It's a feeling of self-empowerment. Our bodies were designed to do it. It is a very creative process. You can't improve on nature.

In order to do it oneself, one must do it without intervention, without drugs. Feminists who believe in natural childbirth are therefore doubly motivated.

A third of the group see the world in gender terms, but not all of them identify with feminism. Efa admits to being 'slightly' feminist. We are not pieces of meat, she says, we are female persons: 'They shouldn't be allowed to get away with it.' Valerie says she considers herself a feminist, 'but not in the "political" sense'. A small number of women within the group reject some, or all, of the current images of feminism. To be a good mother, Frances said, comes before everything else. For these women, being a 'good' mother means making your children your career. Cynthia says she does not share feminist views on the rearing of children or on working outside the home. The issue of childrearing seems to be the core of the issue. Jacqueline, a Muslim, says she believes in equality, but not in '*damaging* equality, in working women and so on . . . I wouldn't be happy with anyone else bringing up my children'. When women analyse the world in terms of gender, and reject feminism, as Jacqueline does, it is because they see feminism as being at variance with their identities as mothers.

In Martina's view, the birth process is what distinguishes women from men:

> Neither can be their true selves when the process of giving birth has been so dehumanized. The male dominates in the maternity hospital. This is not as it should be.

Women should be able to give birth as nature intended, Martina says, with dignity and in peace. According to Jacqueline, there are *natural* roles for men and women. Can the view that, for women, not only is birth a natural function but also that caring for one's child is a natural *role*, be reconciled with feminism? Asked about her political beliefs, Cecilia says she is a feminist in the 'proper' sense, 'not anti-men'. Like others, she distances herself from what she sees as 'radical' feminists who 'hate' men. What is a feminist in the 'proper' sense? Geraldine, defining herself as a 'female' feminist, is of the opinion that some feminists deny their femaleness. And Ute goes so far as to say that she believes in the superiority of women, in matriarchy.

This notion of female feminism, which is clearly related to the female power to bear children, is an on-going theme. It seems as though women who have chosen motherhood as a way of life, staying at home, full-time, to look after their children, need to redefine feminism to fit their needs as mothers, and as men's partners. For them home birth is part of this redefinition.[72] Sue is of the opinion that men are very clinical in their approach to birth: 'It is not the way to cope with a natural body event. Birth is not logical.' Geraldine contrasts what she sees as 'female' qualities with 'male' obstetrics: 'Birth is unorderly, creative, intuitive. But there's this male, controlling, computer thing.' Obstetricians, according to her, are robbing women of the thing they envy themselves, the creative, intuitive impulses:

> That's why a revolution in birth is so important. It would unlock the feminine in men. Obstetricians are all very caring. They have this patriarchal attitude, a misguided compassion, that they will take care of it all. It disempowers women.

Ursula names this new face of feminism:

> What do they call it, second wave feminism? It's part of New Age philosophy. It is a new kind of feminism, deeper, more earthy. It's a whole new way of relating to people. It's to do with alternative lifestyles, alternative forms of healing, taking responsibility for oneself, trusting one's own being.

'Second wave feminism' seems to emphasize and polarize the differences between the sexes, with women as life-givers and earth-mothers. Not only does 'female' feminism incorporate motherhood, it is rooted in the idea of biological maternity. 'New wave feminism' redefines women as mothers, women as power, the power of life itself.

So, home birth is above all a modern idea, not some leftover from the 1950s. It has become enmeshed with other contemporary ideas about health, women and self-determination. It is an expression of natural childbirth, and of alternative health, part of a reassessment of health and medicine in women's lives. And it is rooted in feminism, one of the major political movements of our time.

Traditions die, and ideas proliferate.

☙ 9 ☙

Nativity

The majority of women in the group were having their first home birth. Would they do it again, with hindsight? In the home versus hospital debate, might alternative birth centres be the answer? What would a maternity service designed by women look like? These are some of the most important questions to consider.

☙

Personal Preferences

You know the way Indian women go off on their own to have their babies? Well, I'd like to go to the end of the garden, if I'd more confidence, to be on my own. Just to have help within walking distance [Laura].

Women who have given birth both at home and in hospital tend to prefer home birth.[1] And women who have experienced a home birth tend to have a subsequent baby at home.[2] Asked where they would have the birth, at home, in a birth centre or in hospital, should they have another baby, 81 per cent say they would make the same decision again. The question did not apply to women – eight per cent – who had had a hysterectomy or been sterilized prior to the interview. There must be many women for whom the idea of a birth centre looks like a happy solution, offering the advantages of both home and hospital, with none of the disadvantages. In an attempt to suggest an alternative to obstetrics, the question referred to a birth centre 'run by midwives and general practitioners'. Within the group, however, this was taken to mean an in-hospital birth centre, and it was not perceived as offering an alternative. A birth centre would not really be any different to a hospital, would it, Betty asks. Lorna believes that home-style birth in hospital is 'like beautyboard. It's not real wood.' Freestanding birth centres, like midwife units, are unknown in Ireland.

In the United States, what they call alternative birth centres (ABCs) have been introduced to provide an in-hospital alternative to the traditional delivery suite. This is a response to consumer demand for more natural, non-interventionist, family-centred birth, to cater for parents who want greater freedom of choice about the birth environment, and the procedures used. Linnea Klee has shown how there is a lot of variation between them, with some units offering natural childbirth, and others offering something much closer to active management.[3] Only seven per cent of the group said that they would choose to go to a birth centre, if they were to have another baby.

Even fewer, four per cent, would opt to go to hospital. Women expressing a preference for hospital or for a birth centre are nearly always concerned with what they see as an increased risk to themselves, or to the baby, at home.

For many, hospital birth, no matter how satisfying, will always be second best. Lelia says she just feels that she is better off at home. She would like to see some statistics on whether home births are safer: 'People are always asking me that question, and I've never had any answers.' On the question of safety, women occasionally appeared to have had a change of attitude. 'After Seán was born,' Sarah says, 'I felt that home deliveries were much safer.' For women who believe in natural childbirth, their experience only reinforced their conviction that birth at home is safer.

Asked whether she could have a 'good' birth in hospital,

Frances replies, 'Yes, provided that I was left alone. They do everything to see to it that it is a confinement. You really are confined!' Occasionally giving 'yes, if' answers like Frances, 31 per cent of the group thought they could have a good birth in hospital. Deborah says that at the time, she just went along with them: 'Now I would make a conscious effort, calmly and quietly, to put my point of view without getting awkward about it.' Other women also make it clear that they would no longer accept the treatment meted out to them in hospital. A few women, ruling out the general run of maternity units, name the one hospital in the country where they would be prepared to give birth.

Florence rules them all out:

Birth is a special time. They take that away from you. They interfere too much. They should leave you to do what you want to do. There ought to be more leeway so that you're not groggy from pethidine, paralysed from the epidural, confused from the gas.

She is far from being alone in her view. A total of 44 per cent of women replied with an adamant no, they could not have a good birth in hospital.

~

Changing Hospital

If they just let women take charge a bit, instead of being this *thing* that carries the baby and pushes it out [Sinéad].

If women had the power to introduce one change, and one change only, this would be it. There are plenty of references in the medical literature to the need for 'patient autonomy'[4]. Tríona suggests that what is needed is a different philosophical approach, 'with women being the ones to make choices and decisions'. She is speaking for four-fifths of the group.

According to Fionnuala, women still feel they are being controlled in hospital: 'It all depends on the midwives who're on when you go in.' Many women want the obstetrical drill to go out the window. Within the group, what women were looking for is nothing more or less than the abolition of the standard packaged delivery.

Women want care which is more individual, more personal. They want to be addressed by their names, for a start. If they choose to do without painkillers, they want active support in labour. As Kieran O'Driscoll recognized,[5] one-to-one care during labour is the key to effective emotional support. The expert in childbirth is the midwife, Tríona points out. Her role, as women see it, is to provide them with that support. Jacintha, a nurses' aide, says that at home, you can build up a relationship, whereas 'in hospital there is a coldness. Nurses can be very kind, but smiles can become routine'. Routine smiles are all that can reasonably be expected from strangers. Women want to be given the opportunity to get to know their midwives – before they go into labour.[6]

Enabling women to get to know their midwives would mean radical changes in the way the maternity services are currently organized. Voicing a suggestion made by a number of women, Betty would like to see teams of midwives, so that the same team could follow you through from start to finish. This would mean, as Aileen explains, 'following you the whole way through your pregnancy, labour, birth and aftercare'. This is an idea which has taken root in Britain, officially. In its 1993 'Changing Childbirth' report on the future of the maternity services,[7] the Department of Health envisages the creation of such teams of midwives, responsible for providing women with all of their care.

After freedom, and personalized care, comes the issue of the environment. Women want an environment that is less clinical. The atmosphere could be lightened, according to Laura, and the back-up still be there. It does not have to be like a prison, Sonja points out: 'You could have some colour, some pictures, some plants.' A room of one's own, large enough for the family, yet secluded enough for birth, is what women seek.

Eileen points out one essential feature of this room: 'You should be able to stay there, instead of being dragged out to a delivery room,' she remarks.

The physical environment dictates to some extent the conduct of labour, as Bianca Lepori, an Italian architect who specializes in designing maternity units, has shown in her book on birth spaces.[8] Women understand this. Ursula wants the room to have chairs and cushions 'so that the delivery position is not dictated by the furniture'. Various replacements for delivery beds are suggested, ranging from birth stools to mattresses on the floor. The room should be designed in such a way, Fay adds, so that 'you could have your baby on the floor, or in water'.

꒰꒱

Moving Birth Out of Big Units

Many women believe that fundamental changes are needed in the overall system of maternity care. The centralized system needs to be replaced, Harriet says: 'It would be far cheaper to have cottage hospitals at local level.' However well or badly the centralized system may work for those in the centre, it does not work at all for those on the periphery. Statia, who lives in the heart of the country, has a fundamental reason for wanting to see small units. From where she lives, it is a good two-hour drive to Dublin, and in between, she says, 'there's nothing'. In a small country where one in every two out-of-hospital births is an emergency delivery, the centralized system is a dubious model.

Women understand some of the implications of scale: they see smaller maternity centres as offering an alternative to obstetrical care.[9] Rachel wants to see smaller units 'of a nursing home type, instead of having patients on a trolley basis'. In a smaller place, Lelia observes, you would have a better chance of knowing the staff. There is also the knowledge that in a large unit where they are delivering 30 babies a day, 'it's difficult for them to regard your baby as special'. The demand for small units is also a demand for personalized care. Penny talks about local units where midwives would be in charge:

> Midwives should have more status. They are able to make decisions and they should be able to make them. They should be able to sort out that low per cent that need specialized care.

Sorting out the low per cent that need specialized care can be done effectively by midwives, even with the limited resources available to them, Dutch obstetricians have concluded.[10]

♫

Seeking Facilities For Home Birth

> The midwives are trained in technology, not in the community. The midwives won't take it on without a doctor, and the doctors are unwilling to take it on because of insurance [Miriam].

Home birth no longer forms part of any known course in midwifery in Ireland. The biggest need, as three-quarters of the group see it, is for midwives with training in community midwifery. In the current free-for-all, any newly-qualified hospital midwife may set up in private practice. There are no standards governing training, or practice, in the community any more.

About half the group would like to see general practitioners providing a back-up service to independent midwives. Again, women see a need for specific training in this area, so that family doctors could play a part in providing community-based maternity services. At the present time, with medical insurers charging in excess of £20,000 per annum for professional indemnity in obstetrics, home births are no longer an option for family doctors in Ireland.

Women are divided over the question of obstetric 'flying squads', those specially equipped and staffed ambulances that maternity hospitals used to send out into the community up until the 1960s. About half of the group see a need for them. Deirdre thinks they are unnecessary: 'If anything is wrong, you go to hospital.' Flying squads are regarded by some obstetricians as a thing of the past,[11] and specially equipped ambulances staffed by paramedics skilled in resuscitation may be a more viable option.

Some women mention the need for hospital back-up, and this is related to their anxiety that, should anything go wrong at home, a woman might not be admitted to hospital (see Chapter 5). In Ireland, community midwives, like general practitioners, have no right of access to hospitals, as they do in the Netherlands.[12] Instead, they depend on the goodwill of individual hospital staff members.

A few women bring up the question of specific equipment for home birth, such as oxygen kits, or incubators. Geraldine feels the equipment is overrated: 'What's a resuscitator? The doctor said to me, I've got enough oxygen in my lungs.' In a country where the services for home birth are almost non-existent, the emphasis is on personnel rather than technology. Getting an oxygen kit is one thing, using it is another.

Some women say they would like to see more postnatal care being provided in the community. Women who give birth in hospital, returning home two or three days after the birth, can expect little by way of back-up, other than a visit from an overworked public health nurse. Postnatal midwifery care in the community does not form part of the maternity services.

There should be a full back-up, according to Aylish, with a woman coming into the house every day after the birth: 'Mothering the mother is a very good idea.' Mindful of the difficulties that beset them in those early days after birth, a number of women want to see maternity home helps being provided. A few are familiar with the Dutch system[13] of maternity nurses' aides. Their function, Sian explains, is to keep a close eye on mother and baby, and to do the cooking and the housework.

How should a home birth service be organized? Local maternity clinics staffed and equipped for home births, and providing a comprehensive maternity service from antenatal to postnatal care, is one solution suggested by a number of women. Again, the setting up of local maternity clinics is something that is envisaged by the Department of Health in Britain for the future.[14] We should have community-based midwifery, Tríona says: 'There should be midwives on the district, with doctors providing a back-up.' It would be much cheaper, she adds: 'The normal delivery in hospital costs up to a thousand pounds.'

The cost of having a baby at home comes up again and again. If she had not been able to pay for a home birth, Dora points out, she could not have had one. The midwives' fees are ludicrous, Fay says. If midwives were to be paid a realistic fee for their services by the state, women say, home birth would be an option for everyone.

Finally, there is the matter of private health insurance. Patricia applied to the Voluntary Health Insurance, the sole company in the State licenced to provide health care insurance, to pay the doctor and the midwife: 'The VHI wrote to me and said that midwifery was not a professional service.' Women want health care insurers to recognize midwifery as an independent profession. Until they do, home birth will remain the most expensive option of all in Ireland.

৵

Good Births

To be able to do it in your own time, Dora says, is what matters. For Deborah, what matters is that it brings emotional fulfilment. For other women, what matters is that it is a family event. For Betty, it is to have someone to talk to. For Olive, it is to be left alone. For almost every woman, it is to be allowed to handle it in her own way, without being unnecessarily interfered with.

Within the group, these are some of the replies to the question, 'What would you consider to be a good birth?'

A good birth? To have the minimum of anxiety, both for the safety of the baby and for your own welfare. Letting the woman have dignity by having some say in what happens. It is to do with dignity, being in charge, being in control of your birthing process [Sian].

A good birth? To be left alone. To have one person or two at most with you, somebody you'd know, or who'd been introduced to you, who wasn't on a shift [Efa].

A good birth? To have comfort, someone caring to look after you. To have your husband there. To have a doctor and a midwife. If you're sensible, you know it's not a joyride. To have back-up, personal attention. Not to be treated as if you had no intelligence [Noelle, a nurse].

A good birth? To be left alone to get on with it. As little fuss as possible. No pulling and poking. No enemas. Shaving, enemas, are degrading. You feel as if you are being taken over. A nurse and a midwife, your husband with you. Left to do your own thing [Laura].

Within the group, the need to have a measure of control over the event emerges as the highest priority. Secondly, women express a need for personalized care during birth, hallmarked by mutual trust and respect, and provided, ideally, by professionals whom they themselves have chosen. Other features of a good birth include freedom from unnecessary intervention, freedom of movement in labour, and freedom from anxiety. Having access to one's partner, to one's other children, and, especially, to one's just-born baby, all remind us that women's stories about birth are about relationships.

❧ 10 ❧

Neap Tide

There is only one birth for every baby, Fionnuala said. And for every woman, she might have added. You may have another baby, but you cannot go back and do it again.

❧

Born Before Arrival

What can women's experiences of home birth in Ireland tell us about birth in general? As a case-study, Irish maternity care is of particular interest. It is an actual, working example of what a national maternity system designed by doctors looks like. Deliveries take place in large, high-technology units. It is a system that leads to BBAs, and to unattended births.

Women in Ireland have far less choice than their European counterparts. The policy of the state is to ensure that all deliveries take place in units with production levels in excess of two thousand births a year. Consultant obstetric care for all women, regardless of the state of their health or pregnancy, is mandatory.[1] Drawn up by consultants,[2] it is a model of care which meets the training and other professional needs of doctors rather better than it meets the emotional and other needs of women. Even thinking about alternative forms of maternity care is difficult. Nobody has ever publicly questioned, for example, why hospitals should be closed to community midwives, and to family doctors.

Looked at nationally, for every planned home birth, there was a BBA, an unplanned emergency delivery. This is higher than Britain, where only a third of out-of-hospital births are unplanned.[3] Some women gave birth on the side of the road, in a car or in an ambulance, en route to hospital. A few were forced to deliver in doctors' surgeries, or in police stations.

The closure of small maternity units is part and parcel of the policy of centralization adopted in the 1960s throughout Europe.[4] Small maternity units do not serve the training needs of obstetricians, anaesthetists, paediatricians, or neonatologists. For years, island women have had to book themselves into guesthouse accommodation on the mainland a couple of weeks before their 'estimated date of delivery'. Nowadays, mainland women are also forced to leave their homes, to be near the nearest high-technology hospital appointed for their delivery. In Ireland as in other countries, there was the same outcry at the closure of small units, to no effect. Now, there is further proof – as though it were needed – that even in a small country with a small population, such as Ireland, for those on the periphery, centralizing birth in large units does not work.

Some women are so reluctant to face hospital that they put off going in until it is too late.[5] We do not know how many out-of-hospital births are 'accidental on purpose'. But even this – the only other possible explanation – is an index of failure, the failure of the state to give women, all women, the kind of maternity service they want.

Allowing a woman to be cared for by her own midwife in hospital would be one way of improving the service. But it cannot be done. Obstetricians are personally liable in law for all medical procedures or treatments performed on hospital patients, either by themselves or by others acting on their behalf. How could a midwife be in charge? In the event of a dead baby, as one public health specialist asked in another context, where would responsibility lie?

༄

Going It Alone

Unattended home births, more than anything else, demonstrate just how far women are prepared to go in their desire to avoid hospital delivery.[6] Faced with having to go to hospital to get a midwife, some women will choose to have a non-attended birth. One in every nine women interviewed made this 'back-up-against-the-wall' choice. Most said it was because they could not get a midwife: none of them could afford to pay private midwifery fees. The state fee to midwives for antenatal care, attendance during labour and postnatal care (home visits for 14 consecutive days) is a vestigial £54.[7] So, for women of all income levels, this means having to pay top-up fees.

Criminal proceedings with regard to unattended births have never been brought in Ireland. However, in England, fathers have been prosecuted for illegal midwifery.[8] In a stand-off between women and the state, outlawing home birth is scarcely a practical proposition. A woman can hardly be restrained from having a baby at home, any more than she can be compelled to give birth in hospital. And, as the Irish experience shows, a hospital-only system does not ensure that all babies get born in hospital.

The gap between supply and demand may widen. The demand for home birth in Ireland may be greater than was previously thought. In a national survey of women's health carried out by the Economic and Social Research Institute,[9] 17 per cent of lower income and 13 per cent of higher income women said they would like to have a home birth.

༄

On the Margins of Maternity Care

In Ireland, to say that home birth is a minority choice would be an understatement. Less than 0.5 per cent of all births take place at home, and only half of these are planned. Finding professional help can be impossible. The pressure to go to hospital is immense. Home birth, like community midwifery, is legal, nevertheless. And women's right to a maternity service at home from the state is enshrined in the 1970 Health Act, an entitlement, denied, more often than not, in practice. As well as leading to unattended births, this denial has led to litigation, where individual women, and men, have attempted, not very successfully, to compel the state to carry out its obligations under the law.[10]

The official fiction is that all babies are born in hospital. The state turns a blind eye. What the Irish experience shows, as much as anything else, is what happens as a result of this 'blindsight'. The failure of the state to recognize independent midwifery has created all sorts of potential problems. Certain safeguards, such as training requirements, are no longer in force. No woman wants to be looked after at home by a newly-qualified hospital midwife, untrained and inexperienced in community work. And certain standards of practice, in the area of postnatal care, for example, are no longer in force.

Independent midwives are entitled to practise, but their position is precarious. They have to work without the right of access to hospital, without flying squads. Calling a paramedic flying squad is possible, but only if a woman has had a heart attack. These days, midwives often practise without medical back-up. Family doctors have all but given up home births, because of the prohibitive cost of professional indemnity against malpractice suits. Midwives have no power to sign a prescription. Finally, they are forced to practise without the security of guidelines which have been enshrined in law. But none of these problems can be addressed, because officially, independent midwifery is deemed not to exist.

Women find themselves being constantly advised to have their baby in hospital, by family doctors, by public health nurses, by hospital midwives. They are made to feel they are putting themselves, and their babies, on the line. Half of the women who contacted their local health board reported discouragement. This discouragement occasionally bordered on bullying. Being asked if you want your baby born dead, for example, is more than discouraging. It is intimidating. The study showed that some women, advised against having a home birth by doctors, simply ignored the advice. A few did without antenatal care, and some went on to have unattended births. Actively discouraging home birth, as a policy, does not work.

ॐ

Revolting Against Packaged Deliveries

Some years ago, an editorial in the *Journal of the American Medical Association* acknowledged that home birth was, in effect, a demand for major changes in childbirth practices.[11] Within the group, three out of four women who decided to give birth at home were motivated by dislike, distrust and fear of hospital. In countries such as Ireland where it no longer forms part of the maternity services, home birth represents a demand by women for alternative forms of maternity care, for greater choice in where and how they give birth. For many women, their determination to give birth at home stemmed as much from a resolution not to go to hospital as from a wish to stay at home. Home birth in Ireland is a rejection by women of the way obstetricians manage birth in hospital.

Listening to women talking about birth, the same feelings were expressed again and again. Feelings of anger, humiliation and shame, borne out of a conviction of their own powerlessness. It was not uncommon to hear of medical procedures being carried out on women in labour without their consent. Being put on a drip to speed up their labour, and finding that they could not cope with the strength and the speed of the contractions, is one grievance women express. A small number of women described how they were injected without their consent, with a painkiller they did not want. Routine birth surgery, being cut with a pair of obstetric scissors, is another grievance that rankles. Catherine says she went off sex for years afterwards, and she did not know why.

Some women complained angrily about the fact that their waters had been broken. Geraldine said it threw her off balance completely in her labour. She felt violated. And when she demanded an explanation from the doctor, she was told these were the 'safety' procedures in force in the hospital. Repeated internal examinations are another source of bitter complaint. Rachel described being rolled over by hospital staff, time and time again, for a rectal examination. It made her feel like a big sow, she said. Birth involves the most intimate, and the most female, areas of women's bodies. Carried out impersonally by male doctors, women found these procedures sexually humiliating.

Many women felt that in hospital, their birth had been taken away from them, that it had ceased to have anything to do with them. Nobody had had a Caesarian section, yet many felt that the baby had been extracted, not born. A number of women had suffered from severe postnatal depression after a previous hospital birth. Deborah was so drugged during labour that she could not remember it afterwards. When she woke up, she said, she wanted to go on with the birth.

These are the worst cases. In Deborah's case, she was subsequently treated with ECT, electric shock treatment, as well as drug therapy. In a home birth group, it is only to be expected that some women will have had bad births in hospital. Maybe their experiences of hospital birth are not representative of women's experiences in Irish maternity hospitals. However, the women interviewed for this study were derived randomly from a national five-year sample of out-of-hospital births in the Republic.

If these are the worst cases, they are by no means the only ones. Over half of the women interviewed had had a bad birth in hospital, and this was a major factor in their decision to stay at home for the birth of this baby. Within the group, the markers for a bad birth, powerlessness, obstetrical intervention, and depersonalized care, were always the same. Regardless of whether women were university graduates, or early school leavers, whether they lived in local authority houses, in exclusive private estates, or in mobile homes, their experiences of hospital birth dovetailed, perfectly.

ॐ

Consent, Autonomy and the Law

Four out of every five women felt they had no choice about their treatment in hospital. Being asked to sign a 'blanket' consent form on admission, consenting to any procedure or intervention during labour that obstetricians may consider necessary, without specifying what these might be, is standard in Irish maternity hospitals. Women found that their consent to specific medical procedures was not necessary. Consent appeared to be a technicality, just to ensure that should the matter come to court, non-consent would not be an issue.

Ethically, this type of blanket consent mechanism is difficult to defend. The principle of informed and voluntary consent to medical treatment has long been upheld as a fundamental ethic in medical practice. It is doubtful that blanket consent forms would meet legal requirements. Consent, in order to be meaningful, has to be full and informed. One of the complaints made by a number of women was that they had not been given the information they needed in labour.

At least one Irish obstetrician believes that non-consenting medical intervention constitutes assault and battery under the law.[12] If a male prisoner were to bring a legal action against the prison authorities on the grounds that he was confined to bed, subjected to anal examinations every two hours, and injected against his will, there would undoubtedly be an outcry. One wonders how a forced amniotomy (Geraldine), a non-consensual injection of pethidine (Helen), or an oxytocin drip administered without permission (Christina), would be defended in court, and on what grounds.

❧

The Caesarian Epidemic

Caesarian section rates in Ireland appear to be rising, just as they are in most countries in the industrialized world. In Britain, there is growing concern about the high overall Caesarian section rate. Wide variations are said to exist between regions, and within them, between hospitals, and within hospitals, between individual obstetricians.[13] Rates of 12 (England) to 14 per cent (Scotland) have been quoted.[14] At least one Irish hospital has attained a Caesarian section rate of 20 per cent,[15] which is the national average in France.[16] National rates are unknown in Ireland, as is the extent of variation, if any, between individual hospitals, as hospitals are not obliged to publish their rates.

One US delivery in four continues to be a Caesarian section, and this rate has remained constant since 1988. In 1990, only Brazil and Puerto Rico had higher rates.[17] In 1988, this particular form of abdominal surgery accounted for almost one million operations in American hospitals.[18] It has been estimated that at least half of these operations are medically unnecessary, and there has been no improvement in infant mortality rates.[19]

Much is known about what has been described as the 'Caesarian epidemic' in the US. Although Caesarian section can be, and indeed *is* a life-saving operation, there is a general tendency to over-estimate its benefits, and to underestimate its hazards. Low income women are more likely to be at risk, but they are least likely to have a Caesarian delivery. The same variation in Caesarian rates between regions, and within them, between hospitals, said to exist in Britain has been documented in the US.[20] Private hospitals have the highest rates.[21] The American woman most likely to have a Caesarian section is aged 35, white, married, living in the North-east or South, has private health insurance, and is attending a private hospital, or alternatively, one which has at least three hundred beds.[22] There is also what is known as the 'physician factor'. Personal Caesarian rates among individual obstetricians vary from 0-50 per cent.[23] In one study, other than having a first baby, the identity of the individual obstetrician was found to be the only factor that increased a woman's chances of having this particular operation, while her risk status as a patient made no difference.[24]

The American experience of Caesarian is instructive in that it illustrates a number of the difficulties in contemporary obstetrics everywhere. The Caesarian rate has increased more than five-fold in the US since 1965. Previous Caesarian, 'dystocia', breech presentation and fetal distress – currently responsible for 80 per cent of all operations – account for more than three-quarters of the rise.[25] The obstetrical maxim of 'once a Caesarian, always a Caesarian' still holds, despite obstetrical guidelines to the contrary.

The belief that there was a danger of rupture from the scar of the previous operation led to the practice of performing repeat Caesarians, a practice first recommended in 1916 which is proving difficult to change. It is now known that repeat Caesarians confer no medical benefit and that, in almost all cases, vaginal birth presents a lower risk to both mother and baby. Repeat Caesarians, however, account for 35 per cent of all operations in the US.[26]

'Dystocia', the next most common indication or reason for Caesarian section, accounts for 30 per cent of all US operations, and a number of these have been attributed to wrong diagnosis.[27] The relative imprecision of the term itself may also be a factor. 'Dystocia' has shifted from its original meaning of physical obstruction to a time-based meaning.[28] 'Dystocia' now has a wide range of meanings, varying from 'difficult', 'prolonged', 'obstructed' or 'abnormal' labour, to 'failure to progress' and 'uterine inertia'.

Questions have also been raised about the accuracy of the diagnosis of fetal distress, which accounts for eight per cent of all Caesarians.[29] In American hospitals, the fetal heart rate is most commonly measured using electronic fetal monitoring. The 'false positive' rate for EFM is estimated at 50 per cent, or more.[30] This means that the interpreter of the printout has a 50:50 chance of getting it wrong. In a national survey of consultant obstetricians in Britain, however, improved fetal monitoring (EFM) was the second most common reason advanced for the rise in British rates[31].

The term 'fetal distress' itself has virtually lost its meaning. Fifty years ago, the limits around the normal fetal heart rate were clear. With the advent of electronic monitoring, there is no longer any consensus regarding the precise definition of fetal distress. From being a clearly defined state, it has become a syndrome.[32]

Finally, breech presentation accounts for just over the same number of operations as 'fetal distress' (10 per cent).[33] However, compared to vaginal breech delivery, the benefits of doing a Caesarian section for breech babies remain, at least in the US, unproven.[34] It has also been pointed out that vaginal breech delivery is feared by many obstetricians, who feel that they lack the necessary skills.[35]

Caesarian section, although markedly safer than it used to be, still involves substantially increased risks to both mother and baby. For the baby, the most common risks are premature delivery and lung disease. For the mother, there is an increase in mortality rates of between 2-4 times compared with vaginal delivery. In the US half of the death rate associated with Caesarian section is attributed to the surgery itself,[36] although in Britain, the number of maternal deaths attributed to the operation is estimated at 40 per cent of the Caesarian total.[37] There is also an increase in morbidity or sickness rates, and these are said to be from 5-10 times greater than from vaginal birth.[38]

In a national survey of consultant obstetricians in Britain, litigation was by far the most common reason advanced for the rise in Caesarian rates.[39] In Ireland, in the wake of the Dunne case,[40] all patients have become possible litigants. The law has become part of the way doctors think about patients. The cost of medical insurance, which is currently in excess of £16,000 per annum, is higher than it is in many other countries. Medical insurers claim that obstetric litigation is the most expensive in Europe, because of higher awards, greater legal costs and a greater number of claims being brought.[41] With the advent of near-universal fetal monitoring in some hospitals, and epidurals on demand, the state should require hospitals to publish their Caesarian rates.

~

Shortening the Pre-set Cycles

Active management, an Irish development 'normalizing the birth experience',[42] has been advanced in the United States as a solution to stem the Caesarian epidemic.[43]

> Progress is assessed, initially, at one hour after admission. Artificial rupture of the membranes is now performed ... Progress is assessed for the second time at two hours after admission. An oxytocin infusion is started unless significant progress – one notional centimetre has been made since the previous examination ... Progress is assessed for the third time at three hours after admission. Further progress is assessed at intervals not exceeding two hours.[44]

Active management shortens the cycles of the pre-set programmes. The woman in labour is told when her baby will be born, and this prediction is apparently accurate, 'give or take half an hour'.[45] A system for first-time mothers, it was developed in the National Maternity Hospital in Dublin in the early 1960s by one of its former Masters, Kieran O'Driscoll. Kieran O'Driscoll's objective, according to Colm O'Herlihy, a consultant attached to the National Maternity Hospital, was to prevent 'prolonged' labour through the early recognition and correction of 'dystocia'.[46] According to O'Driscoll's successor, Declan Meagher, it was also to give consultant obstetricians a role in each and every woman's labour, not just complicated ones.[47] Among the claims that have been made for active management are the elimination of 'prolonged' labour, a 'dramatic' decline in forceps and vacuum deliveries, a reduction in pain relief requirements – until the advent of epidurals – and, finally, a low Caesarian section rate.[48] Active management is widely regarded as Dublin's contribution to modern obstetrics.

Now in its third edition, *Active Management of Labor* is one of the standard texts in obstetrics. The National Maternity Hospital has continued to specialize in this approach to obstetrics, and provides training courses to obstetricians and midwives from all over the world. Active management is said to have been successfully implemented in Chile, Singapore, England and Nigeria, as well as Canada and the United States.[49]

Initially lauded in the US on the grounds that it was believed to result in lower Caesarian section rates, active management has been criticized on the basis that it causes increased pain, discomfort and stress to women,[50] that it is the means whereby medicine continues to control childbirth,[51] and that it is founded on an unproven assumption, namely inefficient 'myometrial' (uterine) activity, allegedly characteristic of first-time mothers.[52]

Active management is a system of obstetrics that appears to be both aggressive and personalized at the same time. It offers the obstetrician total control over labour while simultaneously offering a woman her own personal 'nurse'. It is a system which, by prohibiting labour in excess of 12 hours, streamlines unit production, an advantage which it explicitly recognizes. Presented to women as a 'philosophy' to enable them to deliver their own babies 'in a reasonable period of time and with dignity',[53] active management has been viewed in Britain as a landmark in what has been described as the 'engineering' of childbirth.[54]

As a model, it has its attractions for obstetricians, for hospital administrators, and for women. For the obstetrician, it removes much of the uncertainty and unpredictability of labour, so far as time is concerned. It gives him the solidity and simplicity of a measure like a ruler or a tape, by which to measure the 'progress' of labour. Women's cervixes are expected to dilate at the rate of one centimetre per hour, and intervention is no longer a matter for decision.

For the hospital administrator, active management is highly cost-effective. Kieran O'Driscoll described the delivery unit as 'the bottleneck in a maternity service through which all the consumers must pass'.[55] The restriction on length of labour acts as a ceiling on midwifery time. It also limits the occupancy of the bed, thereby reducing costs. One of the basic concepts in calculating hospital costs is the concept of the bed-night.

In offering women personalized care, with their very own 'nurse', active management appears to give women what they want. However, the nurse (a student midwife) is a stranger to the woman giving birth, and once her shift comes to an end, she will be replaced by another stranger. And in other units where the Dublin model has been introduced, such as Northwick Park Hospital, Middlesex, in England, one-to-one care,[56] a cornerstone of the Holles Street system, is not provided.

As a model in obstetrics, active management manages both to emphasize the role of the midwife and to undermine it. In offering a woman one-to-one care from a midwife who has been personally assigned to her for the duration of her labour, active management acknowledges the 'real value' of having 'a personal nurse'. In designating midwives as 'nurses' or as 'nurse-midwives', however, active management refuses to recognize midwifery as an autonomous profession. More importantly, by substituting universal pre-set programmes for individual clinical decisions, it obliges midwives to act as consultants' handmaidens.

As a system, it is associated with a low Caesarian section rate. However, the National Maternity Hospital in Dublin has recently relaxed its rules on epidural anaesthesia, and the long-term effect of this change in hospital policy is unknown. In the US, the apparently low Caesarian section rate is widely perceived as one of the system's most potent attractions. Active management is currently being introduced into a number of American hospitals. However, a major study carried out by Harvard Medical School failed to provide any evidence that active management would stem the Caesarian tide. A four million dollar randomized controlled trial in Brigham and Women's Hospital in Boston concluded that importing the model did little or nothing to lower the prevailing Caesarian section rates.[57] Patients' views as to the merits or demerits of active management were not solicited.

Without active management, obstetric intervention remains ad hoc. The details of the pre-set programmes vary from hospital to hospital, and within hospitals, from obstetrician to obstetrician. Some of the cycles are shorter, some longer. Vaginal or rectal examinations, for example, may be carried out at two, three, or four-hourly intervals, depending on the obstetrician in charge. The genius of active management has been to take this hit-and-miss scenario, and to standardize it. Standardization, it has been observed, is part of industrialization. Active management is a highly regulatory and extremely seductive model, with women in labour as the means of production, a model where ideas of informed consent and patient autonomy appear to have little place. One cannot run a production system based on an optional production process.

☙

Reassessing the Risks

When the United Nations Children's Fund (UNICEF) published their league tables in 1993,[58] Ireland was headlined in the national press as the safest country in the world in which to have a baby. This has now become a 'fact', quoted by pro-life activists, public servants, and obstetricians. In the UNICEF report, Ireland, with a maternal death rate of two per hundred thousand, topped the league for industrialized countries. Department of Health figures, however, give a maternal death rate for the year in question (1990) of four per hundred thousand,[59] a rate which would have pushed Ireland into seventh place in the league. Not long after the league tables were published, yet another rate for maternal mortality in Ireland was quoted, this time at a public lecture on obstetrics in a Dublin maternity hospital.[60] One woman in every ten thousand (or ten women in every hundred thousand) dies in pregnancy and childbirth, the audience was told. Such curious discrepancies suggest that publicly quoted statistics need to be treated with particular caution.

Apart from considering the context in which statistics are used, there are other difficulties to be taken into account. Some of the problems inherent in perinatal statistics have been identified in the medical literature. Comparing the perinatal statistics of different countries is risky, because of important differences in the way the baseline information is collected. In order to be meaningful, like must be compared with like. There is no universal agreement as to what constitutes life and death in infancy. Different countries use different measures of gestation (the age of the fetus in weeks) and of birthweight, so that what constitutes 'live birth' and 'fetal death' varies from country to country.[61] Comparing the perinatal statistics of different years within a single country can be equally misleading, as the definition of perinatal mortality changes over time.[62] Finally, mortality rates may simply be inaccurate: in Amsterdam, where the registration of infant deaths was studied, they found that 14 per cent of infant or perinatal deaths had not been registered.[63] The Irish Republic has only just begun to register stillbirths, and the impact of non-registration on infant death rates published in earlier years has not been quantified.

This brings us to the vexed question of home births. Although the statistical picture is very different in either case,[64] national statistics rarely, if ever, distinguish between planned and unplanned home births.[65] Retrospective studies of home birth, like the one on which this book is based, are the most common, and they, too, are of limited use. They cannot accommodate women developing complications during pregnancy who are referred to specialist care,[66] nor women developing complications during labour who are transferred to hospital. Prospective studies like the one undertaken in the Amsterdam suburb of Wormerveer[67] are much more useful. Finally, the vast majority of studies, unlike this one, are based on a single professional practice, and this limits their value.

Can home birth really be safe in one country (The Netherlands) and dangerous in another (Ireland)? Geoffrey Chamberlain, the British obstetrician, has stated that, in all probability, any 'low-risk' woman could give birth equally well in any setting.[68] On the subject of risk, a random sample of 138 women, even if it is nationally representative, cannot allow us to conclude that home birth is safe for women in Ireland. The study is too small. Nonetheless, the results coming, as they did, from a group who were not all 'low-risk', and whose circumstances sometimes bordered on adverse, are far from discouraging. Labour complications were few and far between, and the percentage of women, and babies, who had to go to hospital was low. The study shows that for these women, the real problems related to inadequate postnatal support, and late diagnosis of babies' congenital problems.

Perceptions of risk in maternity care are slowly changing. It is becoming less easy to view hospital birth as intrinsically safe, and more difficult to regard home birth as inherently dangerous. Much of the public opposition to high-technology obstetrics has come from the consumer movement in health care.[69] Among women who believe in natural childbirth there is a belief that home birth is actually safer than hospital birth. Marjorie Tew, the British statistician, has argued that higher perinatal mortality rates in maternity hospitals cannot be accounted for by the excess of high-risk women in hospital. Re-analysing unpublished data from the British Births 1970 survey, she showed that at every level of predicted risk, perinatal mortality rates were higher for hospital deliveries than for births booked for general practitioner units or at home.[70] Although the infant death rate was more than twice as high in hospital for 'very low-risk' women, according to Tew's analysis, the disparity was even wider at the low, moderate and high risk levels.

༄

Re-examining Obstetric Wisdom

Geraldine identified the difference between average and normal as one of the key questions in the way doctors manage birth. You might not be average, she said, but you could still be normal. In many hospitals, for labour to be considered 'normal', 12 hours is the limit. Under active management, every woman not close to an 'easy vaginal delivery' after 12 hours is operated on.[71] Why not 11 hours, or 13? American obstetricians decided that what was outside the limits of 'average', statistically, must also be outside the limits of 'normal', physiologically. The 12-hour limit is based on the graph known as Friedman's curve.[72] However, since Friedman studied the length of labour in hospital, he could hardly have been in a position to solve the mystery of when labour begins. For women whose labours are not induced, labour usually begins outside a hospital. There is no obstetrically defined starting-point, and significant differences in the way labour is diagnosed in Dublin and in the US have been identified.[73]

Active management has 'solved' this problem, however. Time spent in labour at home is disregarded by hospital staff. To be in labour and not to be in a labour unit is medically inadmissible. To be in a labour unit and not be in labour is equally inadmissible. Even if it is all a mistake, and you are not in labour at all, time spent in the unit *is* labour. Such anomalies, the authors of *Active Management* conclude, in an Alice in Wonderland deduction, 'demonstrate the extent to which duration of labour is synonymous with time spent in the delivery unit'.[74]

Obstetricians claim to have significantly shortened women's labour over the past 25 years.[75] Many women leave it until the eleventh hour to go to hospital, in order to avoid the obstetrical procedures. How can anything be known, 'scientifically', about the duration of labour? Friedman's sample did not exclude women whose labour had been accelerated by oxytocin, or operative delivery, or perhaps prolonged by caudal anaesthesia.[76] Is it possible that Friedman's statistical averages, which underpin the obstetrical management of labour, correspond to nothing more than an institutional fiction masquerading as empirical science? The invisibility of women in labour, or what Ann Oakley has called the exclusion of women from what is known about obstetric practices, has consequences for the very foundations of obstetric knowledge.

In obstetrics, as in every other field, the goalposts of what is known keep moving. Fashions in obstetrics that have largely been discredited include shaving women's pubic hair, and giving them enemas. Now considered to be neanderthal in the West, these practices are still standard in many hospitals in Eastern Europe.[77] Routine episiotomy is beginning to suffer the same fate.[78]

Epidural anaesthesia is a good example of some of the current difficulties. Anaesthetists and obstetricians are divided over the risks attaching to its use in labour. Although a consensus, at least in Dublin, is beginning to develop on the likelihood of long-term back pain, there is no agreement on the precise risk of forceps delivery or Caesarian section. The possibility that there may be other risks, such as incontinence, persistent headaches, aches and pains or haemorrhoids, is not acknowledged by anaesthetists.[79] It is difficult to see any anaesthetist concurring with Frederick Frigoletto's view that, for 'low-risk' women, having an epidural multiplies by four their chances of having a Caesarian section.[80] The jury is still out, to use a legal phrase often heard in medical circles. It is a phrase that encapsulates a serious problem. What is the relationship which is presumed to exist between scientific enquiry and medical practice? And how does it operate?

With epidural rates in excess of 80 per cent in some hospitals, and still rising, what can they do, doctors ask, in the face of consumer demand? Nobody claims to know why the demand for epidurals has risen so dramatically, yet birth by epidural is simply the newest version of delivery under anaesthetic. Since the introduction of ether, first used in the US by physicians in childbirth in 1842,[81] women have looked for some form of anaesthetic in childbirth. The demand for epidurals has been linked to obstetric practices associated with active management, such as amniotomy and the administration of oxytocin.[82] Faced with the apparatus of birth, the monitors and the wires, shutting off the body may seem to be the optimal solution. In some British and Irish hospitals, oxytocin is now used in 40-45 per cent of labours.[83] Have obstetricians themselves created the need for epidurals?

Do doctors inform women that they will have to be confined to bed with a catheter, that their chances of having a forceps or Caesarian delivery are increased, and that they may end up with long-term back problems? Do they explain that epidural anaesthesia cannot be guaranteed to provide effective pain relief?[84] They do not have time, doctors say, to go into the fine print. The greater use of epidural, it has been said, has made it possible to increase the speed of labour.[85] Do women understand that in choosing an epidural, they are also opting for a packaged delivery? The debate over natural childbirth has obscured the issue of power in maternity care. The relief of pain is also the control of labour.[86] Within this perspective, birth by epidural becomes the penultimate stage of women's withdrawal from maternity.

The issue of power extends to knowledge and understanding. The medical model of pain is rooted in the mind-body split, in the body without a head.[87] A woman can expect one hundred pains during the course of a first labour of average duration, the authors of *Active Management* tell us.[88] Within the group, no one described their labour in these terms. Their experience tells us that the body has a head. It reminds us of the relationship between pain, anxiety and control: the less the control, the greater the pain. The pain of humiliation, for example, sexual or otherwise, is not widely acknowledged in obstetrics, nor is the possibility that it could form part of what is generally regarded as 'pain' in childbirth often addressed.

ॐ

Moving Backwards in Order to Go Forward

Part of the problem with the Irish model of maternity care lies in the domination of obstetrics. It lies in the triangular hierarchy of a high-technology hospital, with a dozen consultants at the top, and thousands of women at the bottom. In British hospitals, the position is not too dissimilar. Medical personnel are organized into 'firms'. Each firm is headed by a consultant, and women are cared for by their consultant's team. Doctors deal with problems and 'normal' deliveries are performed by midwives.[89] In many hospitals, unit policies are becoming more common. In a national survey of different practice settings in Britain, the medical take-over of decision-making in the management of normal pregnancy, labour, and postnatal care was documented in detail.[90]

For historical reasons yet to be fully established, midwifery in Ireland, since its regulation at the beginning of this century, has never succeeded in establishing itself as an independent profession.[91] Midwives have no independent professional board: midwifery is regulated by An Bord Altranais, the state nursing board. In the past, midwives had a statutory subcommittee of their own, but even that has fallen into abeyance. Midwives have no independent professional association: their interests are represented by the nurses' union. There is no direct entry to the profession: midwifery is restricted to qualified nurses, and graduate training is unavailable.

Midwifery care remains the only alternative to obstetrical management. In high-technology hospitals, the dominant hospital culture is what influences professional practice. In an environment serving both 'high' and 'low' risk women, the management applied to those at 'high' risk will spill over into the care of the majority.[92] A comparison of intervention rates in a freestanding maternity centre and a university hospital, to take one example, showed that in the case of seven different obstetric procedures, all were performed much more often at the university hospital.[93] In addition to the dominant hospital culture, there is the dominant professional culture to be taken into account. A Dutch study, which examined the neurological outcomes in babies delivered by different professional groups, found that obstetricians had the highest rates of intervention, double to quadruple those of midwives.[94] Finally, intervention rates among individual practitioners are beginning to be measured. The results, particularly in the case of Caesarian section, are not reassuring.

In Britain the idea of midwife-led maternity care, giving women an option of booking an individual midwife in hospital, at home or elsewhere, is slowly gaining ground. What began as a House of Commons initiative has culminated in a Department of Health report,[95] which, if implemented, will have the effect of transforming maternity care as we know it, from a centralized model of hospital care and obstetrical management, to a decentralized model of community and midwifery care, to be provided in a variety of settings.

In Canada, in 1991, Ontario became the first state in modern times to establish midwifery as an independent, self-regulating profession.[96] In Ireland, midwives cannot give pethidine without a doctor's signature.

As far back as 1988, the European Parliament proposed a Charter on the Rights of Women in Childbirth.[97] Two of the rights contained in the charter are of particular interest. One is the right to natural childbirth, meaning 'that the moment of childbirth should neither be brought forward nor delayed, unless . . . strictly necessary'. The second is the entitlement to proper health care 'if the woman concerned chooses to give birth at home'. Interestingly enough, it is the rise in Caesarian sections in the member states, and the recognition that some of them are unnecessary, which provided the impetus for the charter. What is even more surprising is the application of the notion of rights to women in childbirth. Twenty years ago, such an idea would have seemed outlandish. Twenty years ago, there were no court-ordered Caesarian sections.[98]

'Mothers are very often consulted,' we are told about Caesarian sections, as though consultation were a bonus.

Obstetricians talk about 'patient choice' as appropriate where there is 'disagreement over options of equal value'. Whose judgement as to what constitutes 'equal' value is to prevail? Maybe we should go a step further, and consider whose definition of 'value' is to be accepted? Women's priorities are not obstetricians', except in a very narrow sense. In the absence of collective goals, in the absence of a common language, in the absence of shared values, how can women proceed?

The more intervention, the more monitoring, the more pain, the more epidurals, the more Caesarians. Within this spiral, the spiral which is driving obstetrics, we are seeing a deadly dance, the waltz of obstetrics with litigation. The more obstetricians intervene in birth, the more birth injuries occur; the more obstetricians get sued, the more they intervene. Taking responsibility could mean ending the waltz.

Home birth reminds us that women can do it in, and out, of hospital, away from the birth machines. Listening to women's stories, birth becomes more ordinary and less frightening. It becomes more down to earth, yet more precious, than we could possibly have imagined.

$\mathcal{S}$ $\mathcal{S}$

References

Preface

1 Sheila Kitzinger, *Ourselves as Mothers*, London: Bantam Books, 1992, pp. 96–9.
2 Sheila Kitzinger, *The Crying Baby*, London: Penguin, 1990.
3 Sheila Kitzinger, *The Year After Childbirth*, Oxford University Press, 1994.
4 Ann Oakley, *Essays on Women, Medicine & Health*, Edinburgh University Press, 1993, p. 172.
5 Rhona Campbell and Alison Macfarlane, *Where To Be Born? The Debate and the Evidence*, 2nd ed, National Perinatal Epidemiology Unit, Oxford, 1994.
6 Rosemary Dodds and Mary Newburn, *Availability of Home Birth*, London: NCT, 1995.
7 'Changing Childbirth, Part 1: Report of the Expert Maternity Group', HMSO, London, 1993.
8 Kieran O'Driscoll, Declan Meagher, Peter Boylan, *Active Management of Labor*, London: Bailliere Tindall, 2nd ed., 1993.

Chapter 1

1 Thanks to Barbara Katz Rothman, the introduction to whose book, *The Tentative Pregnancy: Prenatal Diagnosis and the Future of Motherhood*, London: Pandora Press, 1988, helped me to solve the problem facing all writers of 'how to begin?'
2 P. McKenna and P. Byrne, 'The changing face of obstetrics'. Paper presented at a public lecture at the Rotunda Hospital, Dublin, March 1994.
3 Carole Mhic Shiomóin, 'A prospective study of 100 first pregnancies and early postnatal adaption, with special reference to the psychological relevance of socio-economic factors', doctoral thesis, Trinity College, 1982, p.46.
4 Mary Georgina Boulton, *On Being a Mother: A Study of Women with Pre-school Children*, London: Tavistock, 1983, pp.1–2.
5 G. Kleiverda, A. M. Steen, I. Anderson, P. E. Treffers and W. Everaerd, 'Place of delivery in The Netherlands: maternal motives and background variables related to preferences for home or hospital confinement', *European Journal of Obstetrics and Gynaecology and Reproductive Biology*, 36 (1–2), July/August 1990.
6 World Health Organization, *Having a Baby in Europe: Public Health in Europe*, 26, Copenhagen: WHO Regional Office for Europe, 1985, p.43.
7 Kieran O'Driscoll, Declan Meagher and Peter Boylan, *Active Management of Labor: The Dublin Experience*, London: Mosby, 1993, p.46.

8 E. L. Shearer, 'Caesarean section: medical benefits and costs', *Social Science and Medicine*, 37 (x), 1993.
9 F. Frigoletto, 'The Boston randomised controlled trial of active management of labor'. Paper presented to the Centenary Scientific Meeting of the National Maternity Hospital, Dublin, March, 1994.
10 E. R. Declerq, 'Public opinion towards midwifery and home birth: an exploratory analysis', *Journal of Nurse-Midwifery*, 28 (3), 1983; T. J. Abernathy and D. M. Lentjes, 'Planned and unplanned home births and hospital births in Calgary, Alberta, 1984–1987', *Public Health Report*, 104 (4), 1989; B. Spurrett, 'Home births and the women's perspective in Australia' (editorial), *Medical Journal of Australia*, 149 (6), September 1988; L. McLean, 'Home birth in New Zealand', *New Zealand Nursing Journal*, July 1980.
11 1970 Health Act, sections 62 and 63, Dublin: Stationery Office.
12 Marie T. O'Connor, 'Women and birth: a national study of intentional home births in Ireland', (unpublished), Dublin: 1992.
13 For an explanation of how 480 babies yielded 138 interviews, see O'Connor, 1992, p. 11.
14 Department of Health, 'Report on Vital Statistics 1990', Dublin: Stationery Office, 1993, p.230.
15 Zachary Johnson, 'Consumer Satisfaction with Maternity Services: A Study in a Dublin Maternity Hospital', Dublin: Eastern Health Board, 1984, p.23.
16 Central Statistics Office, personal communication.
17 Boulton, 1983, p.1: the rate is 80 per cent.
18 Central Statistics Office, personal communication. The total fertility rate has fallen from 3.87 in 1970 to 1.93 in 1993.
19 Jo Murphy-Lawless, 'A lexicon of the female body according to obstetrical discourse', doctoral thesis, Trinity College, Dublin; Ann Byrne-Lynch, 'Psychological aspects of childbirth', doctoral thesis, University College, Cork, 1995.
20 Brendan Hensey, *The Health Services of Ireland*, Dublin: Institute of Public Administration, 1988; Ruth Barrington, *Health, Medicine and Politics in Ireland 1900–1970*, Dublin: Institute of Public Administration, 1987.
21 Noel Browne, *Against The Tide*, Dublin: Gill and MacMillan, 1986.
22 Brenda Knox, 'The role of the midwife in primary health care in Ireland', bachelor's dissertation, Dublin: Institute of Public Administration, 1992, p.3.
23 Knox, 1992, p.4.
24 William Ray Arney, *Power and the Profession of Obstetrics*, Chicago and London: Chicago University Press, 1982, p.37.
25 Knox, 1992, p.7.
26 Knox, 1992, p.10.
27 Knox, 1992, p.9.
28 Adrienne Rich, *Of Woman Born: Motherhood as Experience and Institution*, London: Virago, 1977, pp.154–5.
29 Knox, 1992, p.22.
30 Jutta Mason, 'Midwifery in Canada', in Sheila Kitzinger, *The Midwife Challenge*, London: Pandora, 1988, p.114.
31 Tony Farmar, *Holles Street, 1894–1994: The National Maternity Hospital – A Centenary History*, Dublin: A & A Farmar, 1994, pp.90–1.
32 Peter Huntingford, 'Obstetric practice: past, present and future', in Sheila Kitzinger and John A. Davis, eds., *The Place of Birth*, Oxford University Press, 1978, p.239; Mason, 1988, p.117.
33 Huntingford, 1978, p.236.
34 Knox, 1992, p.26.
35 An Roinn Sláinte, 'Tuarascáil ar Staidreamh Beatha' (Report on Vital Statistics), Dublin: Stationery Office, 1969, p.6.

36 Knox, 1992, p.14.
37 Arney, 1982, p.127–8.
38 Department of Health, 'Health Care for Mothers and Infants: A Review of the Maternity and Infant Care Scheme', 1980, Appendices 6 and 7, p.118–123.
39 Knox, 1992, p.10.
40 Eileen Kane, *The Last Place God Made: Traditional Economy and New Industry in Rural Ireland*, Connecticut: Human Relations Area Files, Inc., 1977.
41 Brenda Power, personal communication.
42 Dr Jim O'Dwyer, personal communication.
43 Department of Health, 1980, p.65.
44 Department of Health, 1980, p.5.
45 Rona Campbell and Alison Macfarlane, 'Recent debate on the place of birth', in Jo Garcia, Robert Kilpatrick and Martin Richards, eds., *The Politics of Maternity Care: Services for Childbearing Women in Twentieth-Century Britain*, Oxford: Clarendon, 1990, p.218.
46 Department of Health, 1980, p.65.
47 Department of Health, 1980, p.66.
48 Department of Health, 1980, p.55.
49 O'Driscoll *et al.*, 1993.
50 E. A. Schwarz, 'The engineering of childbirth: a new obstetric programme as reflected in British obstetric textbooks, 1960–1980', in Garcia *et al.*, 1990, p.56.
51 Schwarz, 1990, p.56.
52 See for example, D. Schneider, 'Planned out-of-hospital births, New Jersey, 1978–1980', *Social Science and Medicine*, 23 (10), 1986; H. Bastian, 'Personal beliefs and alternative childbirth choices: a survey of 552 women who planned to give birth at home', *Birth*, 20 (4), December 1993.
53 Mary Daly, *Women and Poverty*, Dublin: Attic Press, 1989, pp.75–6.
54 Kleiverda *et al.*, 1990.
55 P. Roubault, 'Bilan de l'Activité de l'Equipe de Millau', Cahier, 1, Millau: Naître à la Maison, 1986, p.13; 20 per cent of requests for home birth come from those working in the health services.
56 Daly, 1989, p.36. Source: Labour Force Survey, Table 7, 1987: the unemployment rate is 14 per cent.
57 Central Statistics Office, 'Ireland Census 86' Vol. 7, *'Occupations'*, Dublin: Stationery Office, 1993. Based of necessity on partners' occupations.

Chapter 2

1 Suzanne Arms, *Immaculate Deception: A New Look at Women and Childbirth*, New York: Bantam, 1977.
2 R. E. Davis-Floyd, 'The technocratic body: American childbirth as cultural expression', *Social Science and Medicine*, 38 (8), 1994.
3 Zachary Johnson, 'Consumer Satisfaction with Maternity Services: A Study in a Dublin Maternity Hospital', Dublin: Eastern Health Board, 1984, p.23.
4 A. Jacoby and A. Cartwright, 'Finding out about the views and experiences of maternity service users', in Jo Garcia, *et al.*, eds., *The Politics of Maternity Care*, Oxford: Clarendon, 1990, p.241.
5 L. McLean, 'Home birth in New Zealand', *New Zealand Nursing Journal*, July 1980; G. Kleiverda *et al.*, 'Place of delivery in The Netherlands: maternal motives and background variables related to preferences for home or hospital confinement', *European Journal of Obstetrics and Gynaecology and Reproductive Biology*, 36 (1–2), July/August 1990.
6 Johnson, 1984, p.14, citing contributor to *The Lancet* in 1961.
7 Ann Oakley, *Women Confined: Towards a Sociology of Childbirth*, Oxford: Martin

References

Robertson, 1980, p.227.

8   In Spanish maternity hospitals, for example, enemas and genital shaving are still the rule. See Estela Bence and Mercedes Serrano Huelves, 'Midwifery in Spain', in Sheila Kitzinger, *The Midwife Challenge*, London: Pandora Press, 1988, p.202.

9   Sheila Kitzinger, *Ourselves As Mothers*, London: Bantam, 1993, p.138.

10 William Ray Arney, *Power and the Profession of Obstetrics*, Chicago and London: Chicago University Press, 1982, p.76.

11 Arney, 1982, p.76.

12 Iain Chalmers, Murray Enkin and Marc Keirse, eds., *A Guide to Effective Maternity Care in Pregnancy and Childbirth*, Oxford University Press, 1989. In one study, 80 per cent of those surveyed said oxytocin made labour more painful, and over half said they would not want it again.

13 For a similar account, see Bence *et al.*, 1988, pp.202–3.

14 Ann Cartwright, *The Dignity of Labour? A Study of Childbearing and Induction*, London: Tavistock, 1979, p. 114.

15 J. Murphy-Lawless, 'The silencing of women in childbirth or let's hear it from Bartholomew and the boys', *Women's Studies International Forum*, 11 (4), 1988.

16 J. R. Reynolds, 'The final fatal blow to routine episiotomy', *Birth*, 20, September 1993.

17 Kitzinger, 1993, p.149.

18 The 'good' patient is a passive patient. See Oakley, 1980, p.227.

19 Information is what some women want most in labour. See Mavis Kirkham, 'Midwives and information-giving during labour', in Sarah Robinson and Ann M. Thompson, eds., *Midwives, Research and Childbirth*, Vol 1, London: Chapman and Hall, 1989.

20 See for example, A. V. Campbell, 'On a principled medical ethic', *Family Practice*, 6 (2), 1989.

21 C. L'Esperance, 'Home birth – a manifestation of aggression?', *Journal of Obstetrical and Gynaecological Nursing*, 227–30, July/August 1979.

22 H. Bastion, 'Confined, managed and delivered: the language of obstetrics', *British Journal of Obstetrics and Gynaecology*, 99, February 1992.

23 Amniotomy and oxytocin have both been identified as contributing to the demand for epidurals. See for example, M. H. Klaus and P. Klaus, 'Prolonged labour', *Mothering*, 72, Fall 1994.

24 L'Esperance, 1979.

25 L'Esperance, 1979.

26 Cited in Johnson, 1984, p.15. Source: Ann Cartwright, *Human Relations in Hospital Care*, London: Routledge and Kegan Paul, 1964.

27 M. Klaus and J. Kennell, *Maternal-Infant Bonding: The Impact of Early Separation or Loss on Family Development*, St Louis: Mosby Co., 1976.

28 *The Irish Times*, 'Laois mother who got wrong baby awarded £35,000', 29 November, 1990.

29 Kieran O'Driscoll *et al.*, *Active Management of Labor*, London: Mosby, 1993, p.92.

30 Barbara Katz Rothman, *In Labor: Women and Power in the Birthplace*, New York: Junction Books, 1982, pp.34–6.

31 O'Driscoll *et al.*, 1993, p.39.

32 Jo Garcia and Sally Garforth, 'Parents and new-born babies in the labour ward', in Garcia *et al.*, 1990, p.176.

33 For a similar observation on how the proximity of other women in labour can cause fear, see Garcia *et al.*, 1990, p.177.

34 P. E. Treffers, M. Eskes, G. Kleiverda and D. van Alten, 'Home births and minimal medical interventions', *Journal of the American Medical Association*, 264 (17), 1990.

Chapter 3

1 T. J. Abernathy *et al.*, 'Planned and unplanned home births and hospital births in Calgary, Alberta, 1984–1987, *Public Health Report*, 104 (4), 1989.
2 C. Flint, 'Delivery at home', *Nursing*, 3 (43), October 1989.
3 See for example, C. Searles, 'The impetus towards home birth', *Journal of Nurse-Midwifery*, 26 (iii), 1981.
4 See, for example, Abernathy *et al.*, 1989.
5 See, for example, J. Cameron, E. S. Chase and S. O'Neal, 'Home birth in Salt Lake County, Utah', *American Journal of Public Health*, 69 (vii), 1979; L. McLean, 'Home birth in New Zealand', *New Zealand Nursing Journal*, July 1980.
6 See, for example, L. Klee, 'Home away from home: The alternative birth center', *Social Science and Medicine*, 23 (i), 1986; I. S. Acheson, S. E. Harris and S. J. Zyzanski, 'Patient selection and outcomes for out-of-hospital births in one family practice'. *Journal of Family Practice*, 31 (2), August 1990.
7 L. Hazell, 'A study of 300 elective home births', *Birth and Family Journal*, 2, 1975; D. Schneider, 'Planned out-of-hospital births, New Jersey, 1978–1980', *Social Science and Medicine*, 23 (10), 1986.
8 See for example, C. L'Esperance, 'Home birth – a manifestation of aggression?', *Journal of Obstetrical and Gynaecological Nursing*, 227–30, July/August 1979; Klee, 1986.
9 D. Buckley, J. Garcia, C. O'Herlihy and J. Stronge, 'Husbands' attendance during labour: attitudes and incidence', *Irish Medical Journal*, 80, March 1987.
10 See for example, M. Moodie, *The Pattern of Maternity Services in The Netherlands*, Department of Health and Social Security, 1977; Cameron *et al.*, 1979.
11 McLean, 1980.
12 Community Physicians, 'Domiciliary Births: A Review', Dublin: Eastern Health Board, 1983, p.48.
13 Adrienne Rich, *Of Woman Born*, London: Virago, 1977, p.115.
14 Frederick Leboyer, *Birth Without Violence*, London: Fontana, 1977.
15 See for example, Searles, 1981.
16 See for example, G. Kleiverda, *et al.*, 'Place of delivery in The Netherlands: maternal motives and background variables related to preferences for home or hospital confinement', *European Journal of Obstetrics and Gynaecology and Reproductive Biology*, 36 (1–2), July/August 1990.
17 Bence *et al.*, 'Midwifery in Spain', in Sheila Kitzinger, *The Midwife Challenge*, London: Pandora Press, 1988, p.207.
18 Doris Haire, 'Drugs in labor and birth', *Childbirth Educator*, Spring 1987; Kieran O'Driscoll, *et al.*, *Active Management of Labor*, London: Mosby, 1993, p.82.
19 Searles, 1981.
20 Abernathy *et al.*, 1989; Acheson, 1990.
21 McLean, 1981.
22 L'Esperance, 1981.
23 Barbara Katz Rothman, *The Tentative Pregnancy*, London: Pandora Press, 1988, p.115.
24 M. H. Klaus *et al.*, *Maternal-Infant Bonding*, St Louis: Mosby, 1976.
25 See for example, McLean, 1981; Abernathy *et al.*, 1989.
26 Grantly Dick-Read, *Childbirth without Fear: The Principles and Practices of Natural Childbirth*, 1st ed., London: Heinemann, 1933.
27 R. E. Davis-Floyd, 'The technocratic body: American childbirth as cultural expression', *Social Science and Medicine*, 38 (8), 1994, identifies this as one of the archetypal home birth beliefs.
28 Davis-Floyd, 1994.
29 Kleiverda, *et al.*, 1990.
30 Mary Georgina Boulton, *On Being a Mother*, London: Tavistock, 1983, p.41.

31 J. M. L. Shearer, 'Five-year prospective study of risk of booking for a home birth in Essex', *British Medical Journal*, 291, 1985.
32 H. P. Verbrugge, 'Maternity Home Help and Home Deliveries', Groningen: Wolters-Noordhoff NV, 1968, Table 2.
33 P. E. Treffers, *et al.*, 'Home births and minimal medicine interventions', *Journal of the American Medical Association*, 264 (17), 1990.
34 C. Sakala, 'Content of care by independent midwives: assistance with pain in labor and birth', *Social Science and Medicine*, 26 (11), 1988.

Chapter 4

1 This is quite usual. See, for example, E. Hosford, 'The home birth movement', *Journal of Nurse-Midwifery*, 21 (3), 1976.
2 1970 Health Act (sections 62 and 63) obliges health boards to provide midwifery and/or GP services free of charge to women.
3 Ann Human versus the Southern Health Board, 1983 on the grounds that the time available to the board in which to find a midwife and a doctor was insufficient, due to the imminent arrival of the baby, Judge Barrington refused to make an order.
4 B. A. Beech, 'Home birth – running the gauntlet', *Midwives' Chronicle and Nursing Notes*, July 1982.
5 For a similar picture of the local hospital as a battle-field, see D. A. Sullivan and R. Weitz, 'Obstacles to the practice of licensed lay midwifery', *Social Science and Medicine*, 19 (11), 1984.
6 Ann Oakley, *Social Support and Motherhood*, Oxford: Blackwell, 1992, p.10.
7 J. Cameron, *et al.*, 'Home birth in Salt Lake County, Utah', *American Journal of Public Health*, 69 (vii), 1979; D. A. Sullivan and R. Beeman, 'Four years' experience with home birth by licensed midwives in Arizona', *American Journal of Public Health*, 73 (vi), 1983.
8 A. Kalpin, 'Prenatal care for women planning home birth' (letter), *Journal of the Canadian Medical Association*, 130, January 1984.
9 C. L'Esperance, 'Home birth – a manifestation of aggression?' *Journal of Obstetrical and Gynaecological Nursing*, 227–30, July/August 1979.
10 British Vegetarian Society, personal communication.
11 C. Sakala, 'Content of care by independent midwives: assistance with pain in labor and birth', *Social Science and Medicine*, 26 (11), 1988.
12 Jacoby *et al.*, 'Finding out about the views and experiences of maternity service users', in Jo Garcia, *et al.*, eds., *The Politics of Maternity Care*, Oxford: Clarendon, 1990, p.248.
13 Waiting time, like the communication deficit, is another archetypal complaint made by women about antenatal care. See for example, Ann Oakley, *The Captured Womb: A History of the Medical Care of Pregnant Women*, Oxford: Basil Blackwell, 1984, p. 245.
14 Yet another familiar complaint. See, for example, Jacoby *et al.*, 1990, p.248.
15 C. Flint, 'Delivery at home', *Nursing*, 3 (43), October 1989.
16 Cameron *et al.*, 1979; Kalpin, 1984.
17 See, for example, Sakala, 1988.
18 Both the *Chicago Police Force Manual* (which contained emergency delivery instructions) and Grantly Dick-Read's *Childbirth Without Fear* formed part of the Home Birth Centre's library.
19 Ina May Gaskin, *Spiritual Midwifery*, Summertown: The Book Publishing Company, 1977; Frederick Leboyer, *Birth Without Violence*, London: Fontana, 1977.
20 See, for example, S. Anderson, G. Bauwens and E. Warner, 'The choice of home birth in a metropolitan county in Arizona', *Journal of Obstetrical and Gynaecological*

Nursing, 41–6, March/April 1978.

21 N. V. Koehler, D. A. Solomon and M. Murphy, 'Outcomes of a rural Sonoma County home birth practice: 1976–1982' *Birth*, 11 (3), 1984.

22 Oakley, 1984 (p. 262) describes antenatal education as 'the ideological programming of women for hospital care'. In relation to some of these courses, deprogramming might be nearer the mark.

23 R. E. Davis-Floyd, 'The technocratic body: American childbirth as cultural expression', *Social Science and Medicine*, 38 (8), 1994.

24 William Ray Arney, *Power and the Profession of Obstetrics*, Chicago and London: Chicago University Press, 1982, p.142.

25 G. Chamberlain, E. Phillip, B. Howlett and K. Masters, *British Births 1970* Vol. 2,*Obstetric Care*, London: Heinemann, 1978, pp. 39–42.

26 Marjorie Tew, *Safer Childbirth? A Critical History of Maternity Care*, London: Chapman and Hall, 1990.

Chapter 5

1 Kieran O'Driscoll, *et al.*, *Active Management of Labor*, London: Mosby, 1993, p.32.

2 S. Inch, *Approaching Birth: Meeting the Challenge of Labour*, London: Green Print, 1989, p.32.

3 In 'The myth of the due date' (*Mothering*, Fall 1994), Diane Korte explains why due dates are less than reliable.

4 Peter Huntingford, 'Obstetric practice: past, present and future', in Sheila Kitzinger and John A. Davis, eds., *The Place of Birth*, Oxford University Press, 1978.

5 William Ray Arney, *Power and the Profession of Obstetrics*, Chicago and London: Chicago University Press, 1982, p.76.

6 See for example, C. Searles, 'The impetus towards home birth', *Journal of Nurse-Midwifery*, 26 (iii), 1981.

7 See, for example, C. Flint, *Sensitive Midwifery*, London: Heinemann, 1987.

8 C. Sakala, 'Content of care by independent midwives: assistance with pain in labor and birth', *Social Science and Medicine*, 26 (11), 1988.

9 Frederick Leboyer, *Birth Without Violence*, London: Fontana, 1977.

10 Adrienne Rich, *Of Woman Born*, London: Virago, 1977. See 'Alienated Labor', pp. 156–85.

11 Rich, 1977, p.157.

12 J. Green, 'Expectations and experiences of pain in labor: findings from a large prospective study', *Birth*, 20 (2), June 1993.

13 Thomas Szasz, *Pain and Pleasure, A Study of Bodily Feelings*, New York: Syracuse University Press, 1988, pp.218–20.

14 *The Beginning of Human Life*, Channel Four, 22 May 1990.

15 M. M. Manning and T. L. Wright, 'Self-efficacy expectancies, outcome expectancies and the persistence of pain control in childbirth', *Journal of Personality and Social Psychology*, 45 (2), 1983.

16 G. Kleiverda, *et al.*, 'Place of delivery in The Netherlands: maternal motives and background variables related to preferences for home or hospital confinement', *European Journal of Obstetrics and Gynaecology and Reproductive Biology*, 36 (1–2), July/August 1990.

17 For a description of the physiology of fear, see Inch, 1989, pp.47–8.

18 O'Driscoll *et al.*, 1993, p.74.

19 Szasz, 1988, pp.243–5.

20 Arney, 1982, p.213, calls this 'one-dimensional pain'.

21 For some of the implications of this idea, see Barbara Katz Rothman, *In Labour*, London: Junction Books, 1982, pp.34–40.

22 O'Driscoll *et al.*, 1993, p.75.

23 For a very similar description, see Inch, 1989, p.44.

24 Szasz, 1988, p.249. Pain and suffering indicate that we are good or trying to be good. Some of the meanings of pain in labour cited by Claude Revault d'Allonnes (*Le Mal Joli, Accouchements et Douleur*, Paris: Plon, 1991, p.312) sound familiar to Western ears: pain as lesson, as trial, as redemption, as rite of passage, as price of sin, as expiation, as exchange, as proof of integrity and of love.

25 For an exploration of pain, see 'Alienated labor', Rich, 1977.

26 For similar strategies, see A. Byrne-Lynch, 'Coping strategies, personal control and childbirth', *The Irish Journal of Psychology*, 12 (ii), 1990.

27 Green, 1993.

28 Penny Simkin, *The Birth Partner*, Boston: The Harvard Common Press, 1989, p.110.

29 Sakala, 1988.

30 Simkin, 1989, p.76.

31 See R. S. Barbour, 'Fathers: the emergence of a new consumer group', in Jo Garcia, *et al.*, *The Politics of Maternity Care*, Oxford: Clarendon Press, 1990, p.210.

32 Sakala, 1988.

33 Feeling in control may be related to 'breathing'. See Byrne-Lynch, 1990.

34 H. Ligtermoet, 'Childbirth', *Australasian Nurses' Journal*, Dec. 1982.

35 Sheila Kitzinger, *Ourselves As Mothers*, London: Bantam Books, 1993.

36 Revault d'Allonnes, 1991, pp.87–106.

37 Szasz, 1988, p.249.

38 P. E. Treffers, *et al.*, 'Home births and minimal medical interventions', *Journal of the American Medical Association*, 264 (17), 1990.

39 J. C. Eisenach, 'Labour pain', *Journal of the International Association for the Study of Pain*, Suppl. 5, S1–S528, Sixth World Congress on Pain, 1990.

40 L. McLean, 'Home birth in New Zealand', *New Zealand Nursing Journal*, July 1980; Sakala, 1988.

41 S. White, 'Planned home birth in Auckland', *New Zealand Nursing Forum*, 10 (1), 1982.

42 J. Cameron, *et al.*, 'Home birth in Salt Lake County, Utah', *American Journal of Public Health*, 69 (vii), 1979.

43 For a view that gas is 'natural', see Green, 1993.

44 Barbara Katz Rothman, 'Midwives in transition: The structure of a clinical revolution', *Social Problems*, 30 (3), February 1983.

45 O'Driscoll *et al.*, 1993, p.51.

46 O'Driscoll *et al.*, 1993, p.33.

47 Simkin, 1992, pp.57–8.

48 Rich, 1977, p.164.

49 For a view of a four-hour second stage as 'normal' see Katz Rothman, 1983.

50 See, for example, N. V. Koehler, *et al.*, 'Outcomes of a rural Sonoma County home birth practice: 1976–1982', *Birth*, 11 (3), 1984; J. M. L. Shearer, 'Five-year prospective study of risk of booking for a home birth in Essex', *British Medical Journal*, 291, 1985.

51 C. M. Begley, 'A comparison of "active" and "physiological" management of the third stage of labour', *Midwifery*, 6, 1990.

52 Begley, 1990.

53 Begley, 1990.

54 White, 1982; D. A. Sullivan and R. Beeman, 'Four years' experience with home birth by licensed midwives in Arizona', *American Journal of Public Health*, 73 (vi), 1983; N. V. Koehler *et al.*, 1984; D. van Alten, M. Eskes and P. E. Treffers, 'Midwifery in The Netherlands. The Wormerveer study: selection, mode of delivery, perinatal mortality and infant morbidity', *British Journal of Obstetrics and Gynaecology*, 96 (6), June 1989.

55 Marie T. O'Connor, 'Women and birth', (unpublished), Dublin, 1992, p.112.

56 This is derived from applying the labour prediction score suggested by Geoffrey Chamberlain *et al.*, in *British Births 1970* Vol. 2, Obstetric Care, London: Heinemann, 1978, pp. 151–4.

57 Department of Health, Report on Vital Statistics 1990, p.43. Dublin: Stationery Office, 1993.

Chapter 6

1 I. S. Anderson, 'Employment and health during pregnancy and new parenthood', University of Utrecht (unpublished).

2 Ann Oakley, *Social Support and Motherhood: The Natural History of a Research Project*, Oxford: Blackwell, 1992, p.256.

3 Oakley, 1992, p.257.

4 E. R. Declerq, 'Out-of-hospital births, U.S., 1978, Birth Weight and Apgar scores as measures of outcome', *Public Health Reports*, 99 (i), 1984.

5 See for example, D. van Alten, *et al.*, 'Midwifery in The Netherlands. The Wormerveer study: selection, mode of delivery, perinatal mortality and infant morbidity', *British Journal of Obstetrics and Gynaecology*, 96 (6), June 1989.

6 R. Campbell, I. MacDonald Davies, R. Macfarlane and V. Beral, 'Home births in England and Wales: perinatal mortality according to intended place of delivery', *British Medical Journal*, 289, 721–4, 1984.

7 See for example, N. V. Koehler, *et al.*, 'Outcomes of a rural Sonoma County home birth practice: 1976–1982', *Birth*, 11 (3), 1984; J. M. L. Shearer, 'Five-year prospective study of risk of booking for a home birth in Essex', *British Medical Journal*, 291, 1985.

8 L. McLean, 'Home birth in New Zealand', *New Zealand Nursing Journal*, July 1980.

9 Ann Oakley, *From Here to Maternity*, London: Penguin, 1979, p.125.

10 van Alten *et al.*, 1989.

11 Oakley, 1992, p.255.

12 van Alten *et al.*, 1989.

13 P. E. Treffers, *et al.*, 'Home births and minimal medical interventions', *Journal of the American Medical Association*, 264 (17), 1990.

14 van Alten *et al.*, 1989.

15 See for example, S. White, 'Planned home birth in Auckland', *New Zealand Nursing Forum*, 10 (1), 1982.

16 M. McSweeney, 'Low rates of breast-feeding in Ireland', *Health Education Bureau News*, Winter/Spring 1987.

17 Department of Health, 'Health Care for Mothers and Infants', 1980, p.98.

18 Dr Celine Naughten, personal communication.

19 Carol Mhic Shiomóin, 'A prospective study of 100 first pregnancies and early postnatal adaption, with special reference to the psychological relevance of socio-economic factors', doctoral thesis, Trinity College, 1982, p.46.

20 A. Oakley, 1992, pp. 277–9.

21 Mhic Shiomóin, 1982, p.45.

22 Mhic Shiomóin, 1982, pp.46–7.

23 Oakley, 1980, p.148.

24 Barbara Katz Rothman, *The Tentative Pregnancy*, London: Pandora Press, 1988.

25 See for example, J. Cameron, *et al.*, 'Home birth in Salt Lake County, Utah', *American Journal of Public Health*, 69 (vii), 1979; Koehler *et al.*, 1984.

26 Cameron *et al.*, 1984.

27 Marie T. O'Connor, 'Women and birth', (unpublished), Dublin, 1992, pp.92 and 112.

Chapter 7

1 Brenda Knox, 'The Role of the Midwife in Primary Health Care in Ireland', bachelor's dissertation, Dublin: Institute of Public Administration, 1992, p.9.

2 Jutta Mason, 'Midwifery in Canada', in Sheila Kitzinger, *The Midwife Challenge*, London: Pandora Press, 1988, p.123; K. J. Peterson, 'Technology as a last resort in home birth: the work of lay midwives', *Social Problems*, 30 (3), February 1983.

3 Ann Oakley, *The Captured Womb*, Oxford: Basil Blackwell, 1984, p. 214.

4 J. Cameron, E. S. Chase and S. O'Neal, 'Home birth in Salt Lake County, Utah', *American Journal of Public Health*, 69 (vii), 1979.

5 A. Kalpin, 'Prenatal care for women planning home birth' (letter), *Journal of the Canadian Medical Association*, 130, January 1984.

6 Mason, 1988, p.129.

7 Ann Oakley and Martin Richards, 'Women's experiences of Caesarian delivery', in Jo Garcia, *et al.*, *The Politics of Maternity Care*, Oxford: Clarendon, 1990, p.186.

8 Oakley, 1984, pp. 252–5.

9 Cameron *et al.*, 1979.

10 G. Kleiverda, *et al.*, 'Place of delivery in The Netherlands: maternal motives and background variables related to preferences for home or hospital confinement', *European Journal of Obstetrics and Gynaecology and Reproductive Biology*, 36 (1–2), July/August 1990.

11 I. M. Gaskin, *Spiritual Midwifery*, Summertown: The Book Publishing Company, 1977.

12 For peer harassment of hospital physicians who support home births, see D. A. Sullivan *et al.*, 'Obstacles to the practice of licensed lay midwifery', *Social Science and Medicine*, 19 (11), 1984.

13 William Ray Arney, *Power and the Profession of Obstetrics*, Chicago and London: Chicago University Press, 1982, p.136.

14 See for example, Douglas G. Wilson Clyne, *A Concise Textbook for Midwives*, London: Faber & Faber, 1971.

15 R. E. Davis-Floyd, 'The technocratic body: American childbirth as cultural expression', *Social Science and Medicine*, 38 (8), 1994.

16 B. Spurrett, 'Home births and the women's perspective in Australia' (editorial), *Medical Journal of Australia*, 149 (6), September 1988.

17 Davis-Floyd, 1994.

18 Davis-Floyd, 1994.

19 Barbara Katz Rothman, *The Tentative Pregnancy*, London: Pandora Press, 1988, p.239.

20 D. van Alten, *et al.*, 'Midwifery in The Netherlands. The Wormerveer study: selection, mode of delivery, perinatal mortality and infant morbidity', *British Journal of Obstetrics and Gynaecology*, 96 (6), June 1989.

21 R. Weitz *et al.*, 'The politics of childbirth: the re-emergence of midwifery in Arizona', *Social Problems*, 33 (3), February 1986.

22 Oakley, 1984, p. 214.

23 Nurses' Act. 1985. Dublin: Stationery Office.

Chapter 8

1 Sheila Kitzinger, *Birth at Home*, Oxford University Press, 1980, p.2.

2 C. Sakala, 'Content of care by independent midwives: assistance with pain in labor and birth', *Social Science and Medicine*, 26 (11), 1988.

3 Sandra Ray, *Ideal Birth*, Berkeley: Celestial Arts, 1986.

4 Frederick Leboyer, *Birth Without Violence*, London: Fontana, 1977.

5 Adrienne Rich, *Of Woman Born*, London: Virago, 1977, p.115.

6 For a wider view of the 'filthy' midwife as part of a near-universal climate of

misogyny surrounding women in childbirth, see Rich, 1977, pp.137–8.

7 Sheila Kitzinger, *Ourselves As Mothers*, London: Bantam Books, 1993, p.170.

8 Grantly Dick-Read, *Childbirth Without Fear*, 3rd ed., London: Heinemann, 1956, p.10.

9 Ann Oakley *et al.*, 'Women's experiences of Caesarian delivery', in Jo Garcia, *et al.*, eds., *The Politics of Maternity Care*, Oxford: Clarendon, 1990, p.189.

10 William Ray Arney, *Power and the Profession of Obstetrics*, Chicago University Press, 1982, p.44. Male physicians in the US were threatened by the existence of the midwife; unlike Britain, midwifery was economically important to all physicians, and there was no Royal College to protect their interests.

11 R. E. Davis-Floyd, 'The technocratic body: American childbirth as cultural expression', *Social Science and Medicine*, 38 (8), 1994. In a 'holistic' model of birth, the safety of the baby and the emotional needs of the mother are the same.

12 Davis-Floyd, 1994: mind and body are 'organically interconnected'.

13 Arney, 1982, (p.8) points out that, from 1890–1945, the 'body as machine' metaphor grew. All births, like all machines, carried with them the potential for breakdown; technology began to replace attendance at birth by midwives: 'In America, "normal" births disappeared along with the female midwife . . . In Britain, men assumed control of the right to designate births normal and abnormal.' At the end of World War II, the body became a system, and pregnancy became a process, the 'normal' course of which was open to influence from other systems, such as the social system.

14 Kieran O'Driscoll, *et al.*, *Active Management of Labor*, London: Mosby, 1993, p.75.

15 It has become difficult to think (or to write) about birth outside the categories (the language) created by obstetrics. The notion of contractions as 'efficient' derives from the idea of the body as a machine.

16 Barbara Katz Rothman, *In Labour*, London: Junction Books, 1982. Grantly Dick-Read, an English obstetrician, is credited with the idea of 'childbirth without fear', which developed in Britain. In the US, it was the idea of 'prepared childbirth' which gained acceptance. According to Rothman (p.90), it posed no threat to the control of birth by American obstetricians. Instead, 'prepared childbirth' prepared women for the realities of hospital birth, substituting psychological for pharmacological control of pain.

17 H. Goer, 'Active management of labor: not the answer to dystocia', *Birth*, 20:2, June 1993. Goer makes the point that women have not been asked which they would opt for.

18 O'Driscoll *et al.*, 1993, p.45, comment that relating 'progress' to passage of time in this way is 'readily intelligible, *even* (my italics) to a lay person'.

19 O'Driscoll *et al.*, 1993, p.52. 'Progress' is *notional* because (p.44), the dilatation of the cervix 'is not susceptible to accurate measurement'.

20 Arney, 1982, p.144.

21 M. H. Klaus and P. H. Klaus, 'Prolonged labour', *Mothering*, 72, Fall 1994.

22 O'Driscoll *et al.*, 1993, p.176.

23 Klaus *et al.*, 1994, see active management procedures increasing women's need for epidurals in labour.

24 O'Driscoll *et al.*, 1993, pp.25 and 56. Parke-Davis (Physicians' Desk Reference, Division of Warner-Lambert Company, Morris Plains, New Jersey, 07950), the American manufacturers of oxytocin observe that 'the response to a given dose of oxytocin is very individualized and depends on the sensitivity of the uterus'. Maternal and fetal deaths have been reported. Parke-Davis recommend electronic fetal monitoring, lest a woman's contractions become too powerful or too prolonged.

25 J. M. Green, 'Expectations and experiences of pain in labor: findings from a large prospective study', *Birth*, 20, (2), June 1993. In a study of over 700 women, two-

thirds wanted drugs kept to a minimum, and a further one-fifth wanted a drug-free labour.

26 World Health Organization, *Having a Baby in Europe: Public Health in Europe*, 26, Copenhagen: WHO Regional Office for Europe, 1985. p.89.

27 Arney, 1982, p.81.

28 See for example, Leena Valvanne, 'The Finnish midwife', in Sheila Kitzinger, *The Midwife Challenge*, London: Pandora Press, 1988, p.223. In Finland in the 1970s, approximately half of all births were induced.

29 Richard Taylor, *Medicine Out Of Control: The Anatomy of a Malignant Technology*, Melbourne: Sun Books, 1979, p.134.

30 Peter Huntingford, 'Obstetric practice: past, present and future', in Sheila Kitzinger and John A. Davis, *The Place of Birth*, Oxford University Press, 1978, p.241, states that in 10 per cent of women having babies, there are good medical reasons for inducing labour. For the rest, 'the indications are doubtful and can certainly be contested'.

31 For a number of studies on these topics, see Iain Chalmers, Murray Enkin and Marc Keirse, eds., *A Guide to Effective Maternity Care in Pregnancy and Childbirth*, Oxford University Press, 1989.

32 Marsden Wagner, *Pursuing The Birth Machine: The Search for Appropriate Birth Technology*, London: ACE Graphics, 1992, p.149.

33 J. E. Drumm, 'Coombe Lying-in Hospital Clinical Report', 1990, p.79. Only 45 per cent of first-time mothers who were induced went on to have an unassisted vaginal delivery; the remainder were delivered by forceps, vacuum or Caesarian section.

34 World Health Organization, 1985, p.89.

35 Arney, 1982, p.99.

36 C. Francombe and W. Savage, 'Caesarian section in Britain and the United States 12% or 24%: is either the right rate?' *Social Science and Medicine*, 37, (x), 1993, found that 80 per cent of obstetricians in Britain use EFM routinely.

37 See for example, D. MacDonald, A. Grant, M. Sheridan-Pereira, P. Boylan and I. Chalmers, 'The Dublin randomized controlled trial of intrapartum fetal heart rate monitoring', *American Journal of Obstetrics and Gynaecology*, 152, 1985.

38 Arney, 1982. p.102, identifies this as the centre of the controversy.

39 Francombe and Savage, 1993, found that this perception is widespread among obstetricians in Britain.

40 World Health Organization, 1985, p.90.

41 Arney, 1982, p.114.

42 E. L. Shearer, 'Caesarean section: medical benefits and costs', *Social Science and Medicine*, 37 (x), 1993.

43 Arney, 1982, p.44.

44 J. G. Hannington-Kiff, 'Overview of obstetric lumbar epidural blocks', *AVMA Medical and Legal Journal*, January 1993, gives a crystal-clear description of the epidural space, the epidural needle, and the epidural catheter through which it is introduced.

45 Christine MacArthur, Margo Lewis and George Knox, *Health After Childbirth*, London: HMSO, 1991.

46 D. O'Keefe, 'Recent advances in pain relief', paper presented to the Centenary Scientific Meeting of the National Maternity Hospital, Dublin, March 1994.

47 Doris Haire, 'Drugs in labor and birth', *Childbirth Educator*, Spring 1987.

48 C. M. Sepkoski, B. M. Lester, G. W. Ostheimer and T. B. Brazelton, 'The effects of maternal epidural anesthesia on neonatal behaviour during the first month', *Developmental Medicine and Child Neurology*, 34, 1992. 'Medicated' babies born to women who had epidural anaesthesia in labour were shown to be less alert, and to have poorer reflexes than 'non-medicated' babies. What is of interest in this small-

scale study is that these differences were found to be dose-dependent.

49 The very titles of the articles, chapters and texts are indicative of the debate within the profession on this topic. See, for example, Gerard W. Ostheimer, 'Fact and fiction regarding obstetric anesthesia', in *Controversies in Obstetric Anesthesia*, American Society of Anesthesiologists Inc., Vol 22, Chapter 17, Philadelphia: J. B. Lippincott & Co, 1994; A. C. Santos and H. Pederson, 'Current controversies in obstetric anesthesia', *Anesthesia and Analgesia*, 78, 1994.

50 O'Driscoll *et al.*, 1993, (p.86), spell out the 'worst case' scenarios associated with epidurals, namely, profound depression of vital centres, collapse of circulation, and death.

51 Santos and Pederson, 1994. Bupivacaine, used since the 1970s for epidural anaesthesia in obstetrics, was implicated in 20 cases of cardiac arrest among women in labour reported to the Food and Drug Administration (FDA) in the US, 16 of which were fatal.

52 N. C. Gleeson, S. M. Gormally, J. J. Morrison and M. O'Regan, 'Instrumental delivery in primiparae', *Irish Medical Journal*, 85 (4), December 1992.

53 J. E. Drumm, Coombe Lying-in Hospital, Dublin, Clinical Report, 1990, p. 84.

54 P. McKenna and P. Byrne. Following a public lecture 'The changing face of obstetrics' at the Rotunda Hospital, Dublin, March, 1994, it was stated that 40–60 per cent of first-time mothers in the hospital having epidurals have a forceps delivery, compared with 20–30 per cent for second and subsequent labours.

55 Santos and Pederson, 1994, conclude that the effects of epidural may vary, depending on the time and extent of the block, the choice and concentration of individual drugs in the anaesthetic cocktail and the delivery position adopted; Ostheimer, 1994. That there is a higher association between operative deliveries and epidural anaesthesia is generally accepted. What is not accepted is that the epidural 'caused' the operative delivery.

56 Frederick Frigoletto, 'The Boston randomised controlled trial of active management of labor'. Paper presented to the Centenary Scientific Meeting of the National Maternity Hospital, Dublin, March, 1994. The complete lack of consensus on this issue between anaesthetists and obstetricians, even within a single medical school, such as Harvard, is remarkable.

57 Oakley and Richards, 1990. What is 'natural' may be synonymous with what one decides oneself.

58 M. S. Tsechkovski, (letter to government agencies, December 1993). According to WHO, ultrasound research shows the possibility of a serious risk (impaired growth) to the baby.

59 Petr Skrabanek and James McCormick, *Follies and Fallacies in Medicine*, Glasgow: Tarragon Press, 1989, p.115.

60 Skrabanek *et al.*, 1989, p.115.

61 J. Cameron, *et al.*, 'Home birth in Salt Lake County, Utah', *American Journal of Public Health*, 69 (vii), 1979; C. L'Esperance, 'Home birth – a manifestation of aggression?' *Journal of Obstetrical and Gynaecological Nursing*, 227–30, July/August 1979.

62 Viera Scheibner, *Vaccine: The Medical Assault on the Immune System*, 178 Govett's Leap Road, Blackheath, NSW 2785, 1994, reviews evidence linking vaccinations, AIDS, and cot deaths.

63 Davis-Floyd, 1994.

64 Arney, 1982, p.24, observes that the 'rational' or 'scientific' approach to childbirth originated in France.

65 Sakala, 1988.

66 Ivan Illich, *Limits to Medicine, Medical Nemesis: The Expropriation of Health*, London: Penguin, 1976.

67 Boston Women's Health Book Collective, *Our Bodies, Ourselves*, New York: Simon & Schuster, 1976.

68 For a question-and-answer approach to the relations between the passenger, the passages and the powers, see Douglas G. Wilson Clyne, *A Concise Textbook for Midwives*, London: Faber & Faber, 1971.

69 A. K. LoCicero, 'Explaining excessive rates of Caesarians and other childbirth interventions: contributions from contemporary theories of gender and psychosocial development', *Social Science and Medicine*, 37 (x), 1993.

70 According to LoCicero, 1993, 75–80 per cent of American obstetricians are men.

71 Davis-Floyd, 1994, in a 'holistic' model of birth, pain is seen as an integral part of labour.

72 Katz Rothman, 1982, pp.94–110. The 'traditionalists' described here have no counterparts within this group.

Chapter 9

1 Rona Campbell and Alison Macfarlane, 'Recent debate on the place of birth', in Jo Garcia *et al.*, eds., *The Politics of Maternity Care*, Oxford: Clarendon, 1990, p.219.

2 See, for example, L. S. Acheson *et al.*, 'Patient selection and outcomes for out-of-hospital births in one family practice', *Journal of Family Practice*, 31 (2), August 1990.

3 L. Klee, 'Home away from home: the alternative birth center', *Social Science and Medicine*, 23 (i), 1986.

4 See for example, D. W. Brock, S. A. Wartman, 'Sounding board: when competent patients make irrational choices', *New England Journal of Medicine*, 322 (22), 1990.

5 Kieran O'Driscoll *et al.*, *Active Management of Labor*, London: Mosby, 1993, p.93.

6 See for example, Susanne Houd, 'Midwives in Denmark', in Sheila Kitzinger, ed., *The Midwife Challenge*, London: Pandora Press, 1991, p.185.

7 Department of Health, 'Changing Childbirth Part 1, Report of the Expert Maternity Group, London: HMSO, 1993, p.70.

8 Bianca Lepori, *La Nascita e i suoi Loughi*, Como: Red Edizione, 1992.

9 Mavis Kirkham, 'Midwives and information-giving during labour', in Sarah Robinson *et al.*, eds., *Midwives, Research and Childbirth*, Vol. 1, London: Chapman & Hall, 1989, p.132. Kirkham demonstrates that who runs the unit may be as significant as its size. In a consultant unit, pleasing the consultant is a priority, and the patient is 'controlled, admitted, processed, delivered and then wheeled out of the ward'.

10 D. van Alten *et al.*, 'Midwifery in The Netherlands. The Wormerveer study: selection, mode of delivery, perinatal mortality and infant morbidity', *British Journal of Obstetrics and Gynaecology*, 96 (6), June 1989.

11 G. Chamberlain, 'The place of birth – striking a balance', *Practitioner*, 232, (1452), July 1988.

12 P. E. Treffers *et al.*, 'Home births and minimal medical interventions', *Journal of the American Medical Association*, 264 (17), 1990.

13 M. Moodie, 'The Pattern of Maternity Services in The Netherlands', Department of Health and Social Security, 1977.

14 Department of Health, 1993, p.25.

Chapter 10

1 Comhairle na n-Ospidéal, 'Development of Hospital Maternity Services: A Discussion Document', Dublin, 1976, pp.11–3. The case was argued on the basis of the special needs of low birthweight babies, and of babies born with congenital problems. Having considered the needs of the low birthweight baby, the report, recognizing that many congenital problems are untreatable, argued that, never-theless, those which are treatable constitute a strong argument for 'confinement

in an appropriately staffed unit'. Finally, and most curiously, the case for obstetric care for all was made on the basis of the dangers inherent in obstetric procedures themselves.

2 Administration Yearbook and Diary, 1995, Dublin: Institute of Public Administration 1995. Under the 1970 Health Act, not less than half of Comhairle na n-Ospidéal must be hospital consultants.

3 R. Campbell, I. *et al.*, 'Home births in England and Wales: perinatal mortality according to intended place of delivery', *British Medical Journal*, 289, 721–4, 1984.

4 For a sketch of similar developments in Finland and Denmark, for example, see Leena Valvanne, 'The Finnish midwife and her renewed challenges', and Susanne Houd, 'Midwives in Denmark', in Sheila Kitzinger, ed., *The Midwife Challenge*, London: Pandora Press, 1991, pp.224 and 179.

5 Rona Campbell's 1984 survey found that of 1,849 BBAs, five per cent were considered to be 'accidental on purpose'.

6 Jutta Mason, 'Midwifery in Canada', in Kitzinger, 1991, p.126, in the wake of what she called the Caesarian 'epidemic', observed a rising number of women giving birth 'unattended by any experienced woman'.

7 Dáil Eireann, Official Report, vol. 11, (6), cols. 1768–1772, 24 October 1991.

8 Ann Oakley, *The Captured Womb*, Oxford: Basil Blackwell, 1984, p. 214.

9 M. Dwyer, 'National Survey on Women's Health Needs', (unpublished), Economic and Social Research Institute. Presented to the Centenary Scientific Meeting of the National Maternity Hospital, Dublin, March 1994.

10 The High Court: Sandra Spruyte and Jeremy Wates versus Southern Health Board, 339/88. The point at issue was whether or not the couple were entitled to the services of a midwife. On appeal, Mr Justice Finlay, whilst ruling that midwifery services could indeed be provided by a registered medical practitioner, reaffirmed women's legal right to a home birth service.

11 W. H. Pearse, 'Home birth' (editorial), *Journal of the American Medical Association*, 241, (x), 1979.

12 J. Drumm, 'Birth, pain relief and birthing positions'. Presented as part of 'It's Only Natural', a series of public lectures at the Coombe Women's Hospital, Dublin, September 1990.

13 Ann Oakley *et al.*, 'Women's experiences of Caesarian delivery', in Jo Garcia, *et al.*, eds., *The Politics of Maternity Care*, Oxford: Clarendon, 1990, p.186.

14 C. Francombe and W. Savage, 'Caesarian section in Britain and the United States 12% or 24%: is either the right rate?', *Social Science and Medicine*, 37 (x), 1993.

15 'Hospital reports major rise in Caesareans', *Irish Medical News*, 28 (ii), 18 July 1994.

16 D. P. Dallay, Director of Obstetrics and Gynaecology, 'Peut-on encore accoucher par voie basse?', *Sages-femmes International*, 3 juillet/aout 1994.

17 E. L. Shearer, 'Caesarean section: medical benefits and costs', *Social Science and Medicine*, 37 (x), 1993.

18 Frederick Frigoletto, 'The Boston randomised controlled trial of active management of labor'. Paper presented to the Centenary Scientific Meeting of the National Maternity Hospital, Dublin, March 1994.

19 Shearer, 1993: the decline in infant mortality began to slow down about the same time as the growth in Caesarian section rates accelerated.

20 Shearer, 1993.

21 Frigoletto, 1994.

22 Shearer, 1993.

23 C. Sakala, 'Midwifery care and out-of-hospital birth settings: how do they reduce unnecessary Caesarian section births?', *Social Science and Medicine*, 37 (x), 1993.

24 Shearer, 1993.

25 Shearer, 1993.

26 Shearer, 1993: repeat Caesarians account for half the rise since 1980.

References

27 Shearer, 1993: one third of the increase since 1980 is due to 'dystocia'.
28 William Ray Arney, *Power and the Profession of Obstetrics*, Chicago and London: The University of Chicago Press, 1982, p.146.
29 Shearer, 1993: the diagnosis is responsible for 16 per cent of the overall rise.
30 Shearer, 1993.
31 Francome and Savage, 1993.
32 Arney, 1982, pp.139–40.
33 Shearer, 1993: breech babies are increasingly delivered by Caesarian section, and this accounts for five per cent of the total growth in rates since 1980.
34 Shearer, 1993.
35 Francombe and Savage, 1993.
36 Shearer, 1993.
37 Francombe and Savage, 1993.
38 Shearer, 1993.
39 Francombe and Savage, 1993.
40 Gene Kerrigan, *Nothing But the Truth*, Dublin: Tomar, 1990. The Dunne case has become legendary in the annals of obstetrics in Ireland. In 1988, Catherine Dunne was awarded over one million pounds (later reduced on appeal) against the National Maternity Hospital in compensation for her son, who suffered major brain damage during a twin delivery. The case was marked by missing midwifery case-notes, a missing midwife, and the rebuttal of expert medical evidence by women who themselves had given birth to twins in the same hospital.
41 C. James, Medical Defense Union Ltd., 'Obstetric and Gynaecological Litigation – the Risk and its Management'. Paper presented to the Centenary Scientific Meeting of the National Maternity Hospital, Dublin, March 1994.
42 M. H. Klaus, J. H. Kennell and P. H. Klaus, 'National Maternity Hospital, Holles Street 1894–1994: 100 Years of Life', Dublin: DBA Publications, 1994, p.2, taken from *Mothering the Mother: How a Doula Can Help You have a Shorter, Easier and Healthier Birth*, M. H. Klaus *et al.*, Reading, MA: Addison-Wesley, 1993. (The doula is the only non-professional member of an obstetric team. Doulas are generally female).
43 W. Fraser, 'Methodologic issues in assessing the active management of labor', Roundtable Discussion: Active Management of Labor – Benefits and Risks, Part II. *Birth*, 20:3, September 1993.
44 Kieran O'Driscoll, *et al.*, *Active Management of Labor*, London: Mosby, 1993, pp.51–2.
45 O'Driscoll *et al.*, 1993, p.46.
46 C. O'Herlihy, 'Active management: a continuous benefit in nulliparous labour', Roundtable Discussion: Active Management of Labor – Benefits and Risks, *Birth*, 20:2, June 1993.
47 D. Meagher, 'The beginnings of active management of labor'. Paper presented to the Centenary Scientific Meeting of the National Maternity Hospital, Dublin, March 1994.
48 O'Herlihy, 1993.
49 O'Herlihy, 1993.
50 H. Goer, 'Active management of labor: not the answer to dystocia', Roundtable Discussion: Active Management of Labor – Benefits and Risks, *Birth*, 20:2, June 1993; Fraser, 1993.
51 K. J. Kaufman, 'Effective control or effective care?', Roundtable Discussion: Active Management of Labor – Benefits and Risks, Part II, *Birth*, 20:3, September 1993.
52 M. J. N. C. Keirse, 'A final comment . . . managing the uterus, the woman, or whom?', Roundtable Discussion: Active Management of Labor – Benefits and Risks, Part II, *Birth*, 20:3, September 1993.
53 Klaus *et al.*, 1994, p.17.

54 E. W. Schwarz, 'The engineering of childbirth: a new obstetric programme as reflected in British obstetric textbooks, 1960–1980', in Garcia *et al.*, 1990, p.56.

55 O'Driscoll *et al.*, 1993, p.114. In the current edition, the word 'mother' replaces 'consumer'.

56 H. Gordon, 'Experience in Northwick Park'. Paper presented to the Centenary Scientific Meeting of the National Maternity Hospital, Dublin, March 1994.

57 Frigoletto, 1994.

58 United Nations Children's Fund (UNICEF), 'The Progress of Nations: The nations of the world ranked according to their achievements in health, nutrition, education, family planning, and progress for women', New York: UNICEF, 1993, p.39.

59 Department of Health, 'Report on Vital Statistics 1990', Dublin: Stationery Office, 1993, p.37.

60 P. McKenna and P. Byrne, 'The changing face of obstetrics'. Paper presented as part of a public lecture at the Rotunda Hospital, Dublin, March 1994.

61 World Health Organization, 'Having a Baby in Europe: Public Health in Europe', 26, Copenhagen: WHO Regional Office for Europe, 1985, pp.58–61.

62 World Health Organization, 1985, p.59.

63 P. E. Treffers, *et al.*, 'Home births and minimal medical interventions', *Journal of the American Medical Association*, 264 (17), 1990. Currently, the term 'infant deaths' in Ireland refers to the deaths of babies under one year, while the term 'perinatal deaths' is used for deaths within one week of birth, as well as stillbirths at or over 28 weeks of pregnancy.

64 R. Campbell *et al.*, 1984. The perinatal mortality rate for planned home births was 4.1 per 1,000, whilst for births booked for a consultant unit which took place at home, it was 67.5.

65 World Health Organization, 1985, p.42.

66 T. J. Abernathy *et al.*, 'Planned and unplanned home births and hospital births in Calgary, Alberta, 1984–1987', Public Health Report, 104 (4), 1989.

67 D. van Alten, *et al.*, 'Midwifery in The Netherlands. The Wormerveer study: selection, mode of delivery, perinatal mortality and infant morbidity', *British Journal of Obstetrics and Gynaecology*, 96 (6), June 1989. Based on an independent midwives' practice, the study included both women who were subsequently referred for consultant care during pregnancy, as well as those who transferred to hospital during labour.

68 G. Chamberlain, 'The place of birth – striking a balance', *Practitioner*, 232, (1452), July 1988.

69 Oakley *et al.*, 1990, p.186.

70 Marjorie Tew, *Safer Childbirth? A Critical History of Maternity Care*, London: Chapman and Hall, 1990, p.255. For a detailed criticism of the risk scores, see Chapter 4. She has also been criticized for not excluding from her analysis deaths from congenital problems. Nevertheless, her work has raised fundamental questions.

71 O'Driscoll *et al.*, 1993, p.35.

72 Far from regarding this as an example of flawed thinking, as some have suggested, Arney, 1982, (p.145) sees the use of the Friedman curve by obstetricians as part of what he calls 'the new order of obstetrical control', subjecting labour to the rule of the labour graph.

73 M. H. Klaus *et al.*, 'Prolonged labour', *Mothering*, 72, Fall 1994.

74 O'Driscoll *et al.*, 1993, p.33.

75 D. Meagher, 'The beginnings of active management of labour'. Paper presented to the Centenary Scientific Meeting of the National Maternity Hospital, Dublin, March 1994.

76 C. Crowther, M. Enkin, M. J. N. C. Keirse and I. Brown, 'Monitoring the progress of labour', in I. Chalmers, M. Enkin and M. J. N. C. Keirse, eds., *Effective*

Care in Pregnancy and Childbirth, Vol 2, Oxford University Press, 1989, p.833.

77 Sheila Kitzinger, *Ourselves As Mothers*, London: Bantam Books, 1993, p.122.

78 J. R. Reynolds, 'The final fatal blow to routine episiotomy', *Birth*, 20, September 1993.

79 Christine MacArthur, *et al.*, *Health After Childbirth*, London: HMSO, 1991. A study of the long term consequences of epidural anaesthesia in 11,701 women found a direct association with epidurals in the case of backache, frequent headaches, and aches and pains. In the case of haemorrhoids or piles, they were associated with longer second stage labours and with forceps deliveries, both of which are associated with epidurals. The picture for stress incontinence is similar. In March 1994, at a meeting of the Royal College of Obstetricians and Gynaecologists, British anaesthetists voted overwhelmingly to reject these findings.

80 Frigoletto, 1994.

81 Arney, 1982, p.44.

82 Klaus *et al.*, 1994.

83 Francombe and Savage, 1993.

84 J. M. Green, 'Expectations and experiences of pain in labor: findings from a large prospective study', *Birth*, 20 (2), June 1993. Only three-quarters of the women who used epidural anaesthesia found it very effective.

85 Peter Huntingford, 'Obstetric practice; past, present and future', in Sheila Kitzinger *et al.*, eds., *The Place of Birth*, Oxford University Press, 1978, p.242.

86 Arney, 1982, (p.44) observes that the use of ether, while eliminating the 'unbearable pains' of childbirth, also eliminated the woman from effective participation in birth, and made necessary 'the attendance by a person skilled in the use of instruments'. Some obstetricians would make the same observation about epidurals.

87 See for example, Arney, 1982, p.210.

88 O'Driscoll *et al.*, 1993, p.74.

89 Francombe and Savage, 1993.

90 Sarah Robinson, 'Maintaining the independence of the midwifery profession: a continuing struggle', in Garcia *et al.*, 1990, p.79.

91 Brenda Knox, 'The role of the midwife in primary health care in Ireland', bachelor's dissertation, Dublin: Institute of Public Administration, 1992, p.10.

92 M. Klein, 'The active management of labor: whose agenda?', *Birth*, 20 (2), June 1993.

93 Klein, 1993.

94 P. E. Treffers *et al.*, 1990. This study, of over 1,000 newborn babies, found that obstetricians performed episiotomies almost twice as frequently as midwives, and used oxytocin four times more often. No difference in neurological outcomes was found.

95 Department of Health, 'Changing Childbirth', Part 1, Report of the Expert Maternity Group, London: HMSO, 1993.

96 Mason, 1991, p.129.

97 European Parliament, Resolution on a Charter on the Rights of Women in Childbirth, A2-38/88, July 1988.

98 B. Hewson, 'Court-ordered Caesarian: ethical triumph, or surgical rape?', *AIMS* (Association for Improvements in the Maternity Services) *Journal*, 6 (2), Summer 1994. In 1992, in London, Bloomsbury and Islington Health Authority were empowered to perform a Caesarian section on a competent adult in labour against her will. Although court-ordered Caesarians have been performed in the US since the 1980s, it was Britain's first. The case took 20 minutes, and the woman, a Nigerian, was not represented. While the American medical profession, in the wake of a recent judgment, has revised its ethical code to prevent forced Caesarians, health authorities and hospital trusts in Britain, according to Hewson,

Index

Index